C000177909

This book is a must-read b

- ✓ You have experienced anxiety

- ✓ You have past traumas that must be healed

- ✓ You are looking for something different to try

- ✓ You are at the end of your tether

- ✓ You have tried everything but nothing works

- ✓ You need to find and build confidence

- ✓ You are looking to change your life

- ✓ You are looking for inner peace and freedom

Dear Marilyn.

Welcome to my world?

Best wishes

Caroline

14/12/22

The Ultimate Innate Solution for Well-Being

FEEL IT TO HEAL IT

Insights into the Power of Letting Go

CAROLINE PURVEY

Foreword by Professor Gordon Turnbull

First published in Great Britain
in 2020 by Book Brilliance Publishing
265A Fir Tree Road, Epsom, Surrey, KT17 3LF
+44 (0)20 8641 5090
www.bookbrilliancepublishing.com
admin@bookbrilliancepublishing.com

© Copyright Caroline Purvey 2020
Psoas muscle, roller-coaster, diamond and Cards illustrated by Jennifer Garrity

The moral right of Caroline Purvey to be identified as the author of
this work has been asserted in accordance with the
Copyright, Designs and Patents Acts 1988.

All rights reserved. No part of this publication may be reproduced, stored in
a retrieval system, or transmitted, in any form or by any means without the
prior written permission of the publisher, nor be otherwise circulated in any
form of binding or cover than that in which it is published and without similar
condition being imposed on the subsequent purchaser.

A CIP catalogue record for this book is available at the British Library.

ISBN 978-1-913770-00-6
Typeset in Garamond
Printed in Great Britain by 4edge Ltd

Every effort has been made to obtain permissions where reference to
copyright is quoted. Apologies for any omissions in this respect. To be assured,
acknowledgements will be made in future editions.

This book is not intended as a substitute for the medical advice of physicians.
The reader should regularly consult a physician in matters relating to
his/her health and particularly with respect to any symptoms that may
require diagnosis or medical attention.

'Cats in the Cradle', words and music by Sandy and Harry Chapin,
is reproduced by kind permission of WC Music Corp.

In loving memory of my parents,
thank you for my life.

To my children and grandchildren,
who are my life and I love dearly.

'A comfort zone is a beautiful place but nothing ever grows there.'

John Assaraf
Philanthropist, global leading behavioural and mindset expert, and author of 'Innercise: The New Science to Unlock Your Brain's Inner Power'

For the Reader

Without the amazing sharing of information and feedback from clients, this book would never have come about. To protect their identities, please be aware many of the names of individuals featured have been changed. This book is an honest reflection of my experiences; there have been no embellishments.

It is important you are aware that due to the powerful nature of what is seemingly a simple practice, there are no instructions in this book for the Total Release Experience® programme. You will find details on how to learn the Total Release Experience® Programme on our website www.treuk.com

Praise for Feel It to Heal It

'This book is more than one woman's journey; it is a reflection of a vision, a mission, and a massive higher purpose and the impact that it has on the lives of all who experience it. It's also just the tip of the iceberg of the lives that the Total Release Experience® will touch upon and transform. I went to a TRE UK® Workshop (before they were available online) because I'd met Caroline and Daniel at an event. As a holistic practitioner, I like to be able to recommend other practices to my clients - but only if I've experienced them and know they work.

I was healthily sceptical. 1) I didn't have any major trauma in my life and they'd spoken about 'releasing trauma' 2) I'd already done a heap of work on my subconscious 'stuff' that had held me back in life 3) I had my own modality that I use and wasn't sure I really needed anything else. I was wrong. I learnt a technique to add to my self-care toolkit, as well as having something else I could recommend to my clients. This book is a fabulous introduction to the power of the Total Release Experience® and its incredibly practical and simple way of releasing the everyday stresses of life (as well as the bigger challenges and traumas). Some of the stories will move you to tears, and hopefully will also get you moving your body in this very special way. Pick it up and pick up the practice, today!'

Judith Quin
Vocal Confidence Specialist & Voice-Vibration Sound Healer, International Public Speaker, Award Winning Coach, Best-Selling Author of *Stop Shoulding, Start Wanting* & Member of the Association of Transformational Leaders Europe

'As a Health and Well-being Champion for an NHS Trust, I am well aware of the impact that the global pandemic has had on all of our physical, mental and emotional well-being. Stress and anxiety levels for NHS staff have dramatically increased, mine included. Current options can be costly, time-consuming and mostly ineffective, at getting to the root cause.

I learned the Total Release Experience® for my own stress management and am quite astounded by the impact it has had for me in lowering my stress levels and building resilience, motivation, and focus.

I am keen that as many people as possible, whom I know must be suffering, get to know there is something out there that works. I am so excited that this book has been written. It comes at a time when I feel many are ready to be more open. We are living in different times and although the impact of stress and anxiety is never going to change, our attitude in how we can deal with it certainly can.

We really do all need to take responsibility for our own well-being. The impact? I think it needs no imagination!'

Dawn Pepin
Senior Radiographer, East Kent Hospitals

༄

'I had the privilege to meet Caroline when I led an expedition of female entrepreneurs to Malawi. The purpose of this trip was to support women in business, grow powerful global collaborations and to focus on their own mental health and well-being.

I had never come across the Total Release Experience® Programme and to be honest I was very sceptical, even when I first experienced it amongst the stunning, breathtakingly beautiful mountains of Mount Mulanje, Malawi. The session was fantastic. I felt so de-stressed afterwards, but at the time I put it down to the beauty of the location, and the amazing women I was with on this trip.

As a Life Coach, I am always one for extending my toolkit of resources. Interestingly, I used every excuse to not make the time to do this myself ... work pressures, commitment, fatigue, you name it, until I hit a brick wall one day when I experienced a major meltdown. My husband decided after 33 years of marriage that he wanted a new life ... without me. The news was totally unexpected and devastating for the whole family. For the first time in my life, I experienced pain, stress and anxiety for the future like I have never experienced before. Not even the train crash I was involved in in the '90s impacted on me in the way the divorce has. It took my stress levels and pain to a totally different level.

It was Caroline's persistence in encouraging me to use her technique which changed my life. I realised how right she was. The technique really has helped me to heal and deal with the whole stressful legal process of divorce and the reality of a new life. When you are in your fifties and you think that your future is secure, to be faced with the realisation that your life is taking an unexpected turn is totally overwhelming.

With Caroline's constant support, I realised, **truly** realised for the very first time, that your wealth is your health. It's something we truly undervalue. That it's very easy to block trauma and keep carrying on when inside you are barely coping, pretending to be strong. Caroline's passion and persistence in sharing her vision is unprecedented. She really is making a real difference in people's lives in sharing her programme. Thank you for this book, Caroline; it has come at a time when the world most needs it.'

Ania Jeffries
Award-winning Coach within Education, *Women Work* Founder, Mentor for The Prince's Trust, Ambassador of *Girl Rising,* Broadcaster, Author, TEDx Speaker.

Caroline Purvey's slap-in-the-face message could not be more powerful or, indeed, more timely. It is that we all hold the key to freeing ourselves of stress, anxiety and trauma in our own hands. Use that key to heal yourself or regret it, she declares.

Almost a decade ago in South Africa, the author discovered a technique that involves 'releasing' and, developed it into a 5-step programme called the Total Release Experience®.

She vowed to share with others her breakthrough insights into the healing power within us, and embarked on a 1,400-mile tour of the UK.

This book, full of illuminating and inspirational testimonies of her clients' positive reaction to the Total Release Experience®, is a potential life changer at a time when physical, mental and emotional issues are dominating news headlines.

The shocking impact of Covid-19 on health workers, carers and other frontline staff, as well as a phalanx of school and university students, is reason enough for leaders throughout society to read and take heed of *Feel It To Heal It*.

Peter Erlam
Freelance Journalist

❧

And From Malawi….

YODEP MALAWI: 'YODEP thanks Caroline for her passion to introduce the activity to our catchment areas of Mindano, Mwambo and Chikowi.'

Joy

❧

'The Release activity helps a lot in our community as we empty our stress buckets. Thank you, Caroline, for being part and parcel of YODEP working together as a team.'

Sarah YODEP

❧

'I cannot forget you anymore, you're special to all of us in Malawi, who are much benefitting from what you shared with us.'

Chiyemkezo

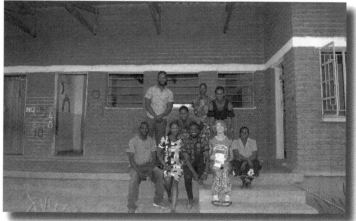

With the YODEP Team in Malawi

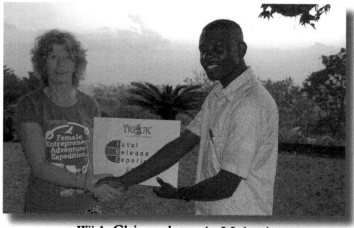

With Chiyemkezo in Malawi

Contents

Chapters Summary

♦ Part I – Setting the Scene

Chapter One: Why This Book and Why Now?
The time has come for a radical review of how we all choose to deal with physical, mental and emotional health. Time to start stepping out of your comfort zone and discover the best kept secret; that your body has the ability to heal. With stress and anxiety forever on the increase, now is the time to start taking responsibility.

Chapter Two: My Story – Awakened Awareness
An introduction to aspects of my life from early year memories and other significant life events that started to shape a path that was moving me in a new direction; one I had never envisaged.

Chapter Three: Synchronicity – By Not So Strange Coincidence
A great believer in synchronicity, the strangest of coincidences led me to the work that has become my life. I made a promise to the UK.

Chapter Four: Square Peg in a Round Hole
Things don't always turn out the way we expect, but maybe that is the way it has to be. But it turns out alright in the end. We might not fit in with everyone else, but perhaps we are not meant to!

♦ Part II – A Calling to Initiate Change

Chapter Five: Stress, Trauma and TRE in Context
Putting stress and trauma in context explaining an overview of the impact it can have on your physical, mental and emotional well-being. An introduction to the psoas muscle, your fight/flight centre, as you get insight into the healing power within you.

Chapter Six: The Healing Power Within, the Inertia of Today's Solutions and Why They Don't Work.

The power of the Psoas and why it is important to be aware of its presence. When stress takes a hold, what strategies you might invariably use either drain you of money, or give brief respite, but never solve the problem. An exploration of a new way of thinking.

Chapter Seven: On Becoming an Expert and a Special Connection
How a visiting yoga student changed my world and my vision started to become a reality. My journey of reaching out to people in the UK was well and truly started. How a special connection came about – so many coincidences that gave me experience I never could have envisaged.

Chapter Eight: Time for Change – The Total Release Experience® and a New Plan of Action!
It's all in a name – what works for one culture doesn't always sit with another. Why language is important if we are to get a message out to the world. Time for change as Daniel joins me – for two heads are better than one as we lay foundations for growth!

Chapter Nine: Diamonds, Buckets and the Downward Spiral – Reframing Stress
Reframing stress with a new language. A simple, effective way to understand the impact of stress not just on your health, but your ability to be the best you can be!

Chapter Ten: The Roller Coaster Ride – Go with the Flow (Feel It to Heal It!)
Riding a Roller Coaster like no other. When Releasing starts, extraordinary change is experienced as clients learn to Feel It to Heal It. Read stories of how blocked tension, emotion, feelings, pain and memories leave the body, setting them free.

♦ **Part III – Taking Responsibility to Discover the Power Within**

Chapter Eleven: Proof of the Pudding – Gary's Story
One man's journey back to health, giving you insight into the power of healing with a regular practice.

With early onset Parkinson's, Gary turned his life around, something he never thought possible.

Chapter Twelve: The Impact of Childhood Trauma – When ACEs are High
Childhood trauma impacts adult health. Sharing the impact of boarding school on Michael and of neglect on Leia as a baby as she endured an abusive childhood.

Chapter Thirteen: Hearing Lost in Childhood – Angharad's story
An incredible story of how a child's hearing was impacted as she tried to cope with parents who shouted constantly.

Chapter Fourteen: What Goes In Has to Come Out – More Insights into the Power of Healing
From phobias and fears, to felt pain, there seems to be no bounds to healing. Enduring years of suffering, they almost gave up any hope. Then they let their body do the talking!

Chapter Fifteen: We Are All Human. Heroes and...
Heroes are those men and women in the service sector that face and absorb the trauma of others on a daily basis. They, like the rest of us, are human – and can only hold back for so long.

Chapter Sixteen: ... and Villains – Setting Prisoners Free!
Taking our Programme into prison was a dream that became a reality. We didn't know from one week to the next what we would experience. Read selected insights and one special story of a life that has changed forever.

Chapter Seventeen: Set Yourself Free – Shine Bright Like a Diamond
Two very different examples of how lives are transformed. Read how Nessie overcame insurmountable challenges and Darren discovered there was more to life after Releasing. They both discovered it is possible to set yourself free of the past and shine like never before.

Chapter Eighteen: Finding Your Truth – Mary's Journey
There are some things you cannot rush. Everybody's journey is different. Mary's is the ultimate journey, for she has persevered to find herself. She is unravelling the deep-held realities of her life where the abuse started when she was a baby – she continues to discover the real truth behind her pain.

Chapter Nineteen: Malawi – Leaving a Footprint

A chance question led me to join 13 other entrepreneurial women on an Expedition/Challenge to Malawi. What happened was more than I could have imagined – I completed the challenge too, but not how I expected!

◆   Part IV – Moving Forward

Chapter Twenty: Breaking the Chains – Setting Our Children Free

Children are our future leaders. They can so easily be shown the way to let go of the baggage from their parents and others, so they do not carry it into their adult life. Can we save them from the struggles of a life on medication, counselling or prevent an early death?

Conclusion: The Price of Ignorance – Changing Mindsets – And a Message to Leaders

Health is our wealth. Ignoring stress and the impact of trauma on your well-being by getting by and saying, 'I am over it' is not enough. It is time to change mindsets, for the problems with physical, mental and emotional health will continue to escalate; it is a global problem. What else do we all have? It is time that leaders start to lead!

The Last Word – A Doctor's Perspective and Her Message to Leaders

Our Doctor is the one person we totally trust and hold in high esteem. How would you feel if your Doctor turned your thinking on its head?

My Gratitude

'If you want to go fast, go alone,
if you want to go far, go together.'

African proverb

So many people over the years have said to me, 'You must write a book.' Indeed, it is something I have always wanted to do. I was encouraged by the fact that so many thought I had something to say! For every year I have said, 'I must write the book,' I was gathering more clients, more experiences, and more insights. I am never one to shy away from change. Just as my work and business have been constantly changing and evolving, so has the world. Never has there been a time to share such an important message as now!

I have so many to thank, for so many reasons.

First and foremost, to the two who have been by my side supporting my Journey which would have sent most giddy. They have been packing my parachute and together we have been a great team.

My eternal gratitude to:

My devoted husband Terry (Mr T) who has looked after me and given me the time and space I needed to develop my work, and to deal with the inevitable or unexpected challenges. He has driven thousands of miles over the years so I can deliver Workshops to clients. His patience and support has allowed me to bring this book to completion.

To my son Daniel, who has inspired me in so many ways. So full of love and support, he has been, and continues to be, a great advocate, practitioner, and driving force in moving me out of my comfort zone to adapt to new systems and structures as we have evolved to create a solid foundation on which to grow and reach out to the world.

To my sister Mary Meehan and nephew Joe Hoare, who never stopped believing in my cause. To my niece Ann-Marie Hawkins, for her love, support and walking boots! To Heidi Stone, for sharing with a friend and opening a surprise door. To Mandy Bostwick, for being my mentor and friend. To Dr. Alison Graham, for being one-of-a-kind, open-minded, trusting, and supportive. To Jennifer Norman, for being open to the need for something else to support school staff and pupils' well-being. To Paul Harris and Brennan Ralls, for being advocates in their determination to drive a message home to those leading their service sector.

To Nessie, for allowing me to witness and support her healing journey, and to Darren, for changing his mind and then becoming a champion advocate. To Mary, who continues her journey showing real courage so we can all understand more. To Ania Jeffries, for the Malawi opportunity that helped me build my global dream. To Joy, Sarah, and Chiyemkezo, and all their teams in Malawi, for their trust and belief in my work.

My sincere gratitude to all I have worked with for being curious enough to want to learn something new and to place their trust in me. Without them, this book would not have been possible.

Each and every one I have met on my journey, family and friends included, that have loved my passion for what I do or have been challenged by it though you may not realise it, you have all given me a reason to keep going to get this book done! Thank you.

To Kris and Jacqueline for advice and guidance in writing. Thank you to my publisher Brenda Dempsey of Book Brilliance Publishing who has been first-class in holding my hand and guiding me through every step of the process! Brenda and her team have demonstrated their professionalism throughout. Olivia Eisinger for her patient and diligent editing, Zara

Thatcher for layout and design, and Jennifer Garrity for the cover design and artwork. Their support and encouragement was always there when I needed it. But most of all, for their belief in my message and encouraging me to get my voice out there and get to fulfil a(nother) long-held dream!

Finally, I am so humbled to have connected with Professor Gordon Turnbull in 2013. Over the years he has given me his continued support and rare opportunities to deepen my knowledge and experience around the implications of trauma on mind and body. I feel blessed that he has written the foreword for this book. It is rare to find one in his field to be so open to the bigger picture when it comes to different approaches to healing from trauma.

**‘Gratitude makes sense of our past,
brings peace for today,
and creates a vision for tomorrow.’**

Melody Beattie
American self-help author

*'You have to leave the city
of your comfort zone
and go into the wilderness
of your intuition.
What you'll discover
will be wonderful.
What you'll discover
is yourself.'*

Alan Alda
*American actor, director, screenwriter,
comedian, and author*

Foreword

On reflection, I think that I've always wanted to be a doctor but I also realise that my interest in specialising in Psychiatry developed as a result of practicing Medicine for several years. These were anything but wasted years and I look back on them as part of my professional and personal evolution. They were exciting, fascinating, and stimulating years and led to the biggest discovery of all. This was twofold: the first challenge was learning how to help people to cope with the psychological and emotional challenges of medical care; the second that a working knowledge of psychiatry is an integral component of all medical specialties and is **never** a separate issue.

I believe that this process of evolution occurs in most fledgling doctors and is **always** essential in delivering effective medicine. Mind-body perspectives **always** shine brighter light onto the more obscure medical conditions and that, in itself, often permits a major step towards resolution.

<u>Never</u> and <u>always</u>

Caroline Purvey has written her latest book, *Feel It to Heal It*, with these factors in mind, demonstrating with great clarity that the same holistic evolution happens in physiotherapists. A moment's reflection will reveal that it will also apply to nurses, technicians and supportive staff in hospitals and medical centres and also to administrative personnel. To emergency service, police, military, prison service and those involved in caring for others in any capacity. The current pandemic, COVID-19, makes that very point.

In this inspirational book, she describes how psychological and emotional dysregulation accompany all medical conditions, and how the resulting *bodily distress* can block the natural resolution and repair of many, if not **all** conditions that we treat.

Never and *always* and *all*

Advances in the neurosciences have facilitated the understanding of how the impact of events is processed in the mind and the body, and new treatment techniques now reflect the implications of neurobiological research.

For example, we now know that most human experience, especially traumatic experience, is processed at a subcortical level, in the unconscious rather than the conscious mind. This finding makes sense of the often-puzzling actions and reactions of traumatised individuals to current, not just past, experience: their emotional dysregulation, their troubled interpersonal relationships, their unconscious re-enactments of old imprinted and trapped traumatic memories. Unfortunately, the higher cortical processes involved in the talking therapies, such as insight and interpretation, often have only a limited impact at best on unprocessed subcortical activity, and therefore, on treatment outcome.

For treatments to be effective, there is a need for therapeutic approaches which address both cortical and subcortical processes. The aims of treatment are to resolve traumatic memories, decrease hyperarousal and chronic impulsivity, eliminate dissociation from somatic and emotional experience, and promote a sense of mastery.

The last point makes a strong case for *Total Release Experience*®. I now leave it to the eloquence of Caroline Purvey's explanations, her experience and her passion for her subject to reveal her ideas and techniques to **all** of us who either practice medicine in all its different forms and **all** of us who receive their treatment (which, by the way, is **all** of us).

Professor Gordon Turnbull, FRCP, FRCPsych
Consultant Psychiatrist and Author of *Trauma: From Lockerbie to 7/7*

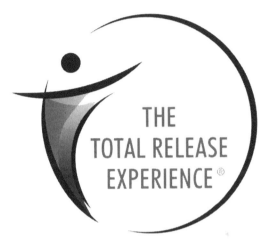

...for natural stress release

'Helping a person will not
necessarily change the world,
but it will change the world
for that person.'

Anon

Introduction

We live in a world where three issues that impact health are spiralling out of control; Mental Health, Obesity and Addictions. It may surprise you, but all these issues arise predominantly from stress. Stress is the biggest problem for us all and yet the least acknowledged. Stress will impact every system in your body if left unmanaged. They say stress is a silent killer, but is it? Or is it that through ignorance and denial you, like millions of others, are slowly killing yourself?

This growing problem is impacting families, communities, and workplaces – in other words, the whole of society. It is a worldwide problem. Ask yourself, where is there a truly stress-free zone? We are all actors on a stage wearing a painted smile, kidding everyone that we are 'OK'!

I personally don't see mental health as being clearly distinct from emotional, spiritual or physical health. We are energy systems that manifest dis-ease in a variety of ways, often simultaneously.

We are told the NHS cannot cope and we all need to look for some self-care. The main solutions offered are talking, prescription drugs, or self-medication. These include a broad range of substances or behaviours that arise out of a desire to avoid pain, improve emotional states, and provide a feeling of bonding that is otherwise lacking. Unless you have deep pockets for self-soothing, often indulgent treatments, then your choices remain limited indeed.

The good news is that there is a solution to your well-being crisis – you can heal yourself; you have just forgotten how! Discover in this book the best kept secret and why you have lost the ability to release your stress instead of holding on to it – thereby exacerbating the root cause of the issues that are catastrophically undermining your health just as they are for the rest of our society.

In 2011, something called me. Extraordinary circumstances led me to South Africa where I joined 99 others from around the world to learn a technique I had never heard of: Trauma Prevention Exercise, to release the impact of trauma on the body. Be careful what you wish for – I vowed on my return to make it happen in the UK. My vision and mission are what has driven me ever since.

As CEO of TRE UK® experience led me to evolve the practice I learned to create the Total Release Experience®, now an empowering 5-Step programme, that directly addresses and heals symptoms from held stress and trauma. It has not only transformed my life but that of thousands of others we have worked with. Our programme is more than just a practice. It is a life tool and a tool for life. It is a practice for life, it is a life saver!

I have been privileged to witness the most amazing and powerful examples of the human body's innate ability to heal itself. Many people I have worked with have shared their stories with me, and I can no longer sit on what I have learnt. I want to tell you that you too have a choice. Transform your life and move from a painful past to a future of freedom just like others have, or take your chance!

This book will enable you to understand what our programme is about through the stories of others' experiences to discover how when you 'Feel It to Heal It' you Heal from your Past and Build Resilience. Discover who you really are when you set yourself free, as your Diamond comes out to Shine.

There will be opportunities throughout with Caroline's Points to Ponder to reflect on your own experiences, to put into perspective your own current state of well-being.

Writing a book was always a dream of mine – but I could never have imagined it would be about something that could potentially change the face of health and well-being on a massive scale. That is what I intend to do. Time now to share with you my knowledge and rich healing stories. But before you join me, I would suggest that you have a notebook and pen to hand so that you can jot down comments as you work through some of the ideas in the book.

'Vision without action is merely a dream.
Action without vision just passes the time.
Vision with action can change the world.'

Joel Arthur Barker
American futurist and author of 'Future Edge'

'Sharing will enrich everyone with more knowledge.'

Ana Monnar
Children's poet and teacher

PART I – SETTING THE SCENE
Chapter One
Why This Book and Why Now?

Why this book indeed? Well that's an easy one! Firstly, because it has never been written before, nor anything like it. 'But it's another book about healing and there are shelves of those,' I hear you say! Indeed, there are, but this book is about self-healing, a concept that is unfamiliar to our thinking. This book is long overdue, and it comes at a time when physical, mental and emotional issues are dominating the news pages more than anything else.

Doctors' surgeries are unable to cope, hospitals are dealing with the fallout, as are prisons and schools. It's not just a UK problem, but a global one. Let's face it, decisions, actions and words all come from the state we might find ourselves in at any given time and depend on what has been going on in our lives that adds pressure.

Yes, that's it, we are all under pressure one way or another and yet we often don't even realise it in ourselves until it is too late. We make irrational decisions, say regrettable things and behave in a way that impacts others, be that family, friends or those who happen to be in our space.

Take the case of a woman who went on holiday with her daughter and on the flight got drunk and propositioned a man sitting with his son. Apart from getting picked up by the police, passengers were impacted, to say nothing of the upset and embarrassment of her daughter. What was the bottom line and the reason for her actions and behaviour? She was still suffering the pain of divorce. Now, that whole embarrassing situation and the realisation in the cold, sober light of day is going to build more tension in her body. Others holding tension from that situation would be the passengers who were disrupted, the airline staff dealing with it, the man she propositioned, and no doubt his son, but worst of all her daughter. She will carry the tension of that episode through to her adult life.

I want to share my journey of discovery with you from working with clients since 2011 and the sharing of stories and experiences of their healing journey. They are not mine to sit on, they need to be shared and heard. Incredible self-healing from a simple practice taught to those who stepped out of their comfort zone by doing something for themselves. We all have choices; they made a choice to change their life and did just that. You too can do the same.

This book is about REAL healing. REAL deep healing, permanent healing, not a case of 'I feel better now' and then years later back it all comes. Because that indicates one was never healed in the first place. Why? Because the tension from stressful, overwhelming, or traumatic incidents that can go back to your early years gets stored in your body's muscle memory, starting deep in the core. Yes, yours, mine and everyone else's. 'So, what?' you might say, 'What's new?'

Of course, plenty of academics have written books on that very subject. Particularly well-known are *The Body Keeps the Score* by Bessel van der Kolk and *When the Body Says NO* by Dr Gabor Maté. They both offer a better understanding of what is going on, including some ideas on what can help heal, but there are no profound answers.

There are plenty of books with proclamations to heal, from affirmations to meditation, but over the years of sharing my knowledge, I have seen many clients spend fortunes on such solutions, hoping that they can be cured of their physical, mental, emotional pain. What many do notice, is that the healing is only temporary. The solution that is going to make a real difference to their physical, mental and emotional health, and that of the nation, requires a real mind shift. Simply this: we ALL have the ability to heal ourselves and take back control of our well-being. The fact is we were born with our own survival kit! We have had the answer all along!

Well-being is Your Responsibility

'If you can't take responsibility for your own well-being, you will never take control of it.'

Jennifer Hudson
Singer

When I first started teaching what I am going to share with you, I used to cut out news articles on stress, anxiety and depression all relative to causes of mental health problems. Recently when having a sort out, I pulled out that very pack and read through them again. I sat back silently and thought in that moment that for all the hype, for all the money that is thrown at it, NHS, charities, services, etc. etc. etc., NOTHING has changed — in fact the problem has just got worse. Why? Because all the while we sit back and wait for someone to do something to us – nothing will ever change.

One of my special and dear clients, whom I have seen transform herself recovering from CPTSD* from years of childhood abuse, once said to me, 'The NHS spent years getting people to use their services and now they cannot cope, they want people to look for another solution.' I recently heard on a BBC News report that 'Doctors' surgeries are under pressure – can we please look for some self-care.' Easy enough to say but after years of relying on someone else to do the job for us, we have switched off to any idea that we can possibly do something for ourselves.

But you can and that is why I have written this book. By the time you have finished this journey, you will understand that you will be able to heal yourself.

* See glossary at the back for the full meaning.

*'You only get one life.
It's actually your duty
to live it as fully as possible.'*

'Me Before You'
Best-selling novel by Jojo Moyes

Chapter Two
My Story – Awakened Awareness

I was blessed to be born into a very loving family; not everyone is. I will come back to this later as it is relevant to the TRE. I had four siblings, three sisters and a brother. I was the second eldest. My earliest memory was when I was around two years old. I was taken to Brook Hospital in Shooters Hill, London, as I had caught bronchopneumonia. I remember standing at a big glass window looking down a corridor seeing my mum and dad walk away. I know I never felt abandoned, but I can look back now, as I have been there too, and felt the pain of having to leave your child in a hospital. Trusting them to the care of others. Rather worse in those days as parents were not allowed to stay like they can today.

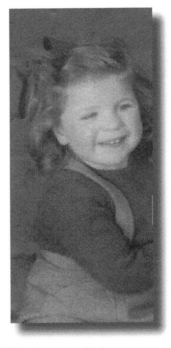

I started school at the age of three and joined my big sister at a little convent called Maryville near where we lived in Erith. I recall some memories of those days too, one in particular. It was lunchtime and we were all sat at the tables in the dining hall. There was a bit of commotion. The nuns rallied around a girl who had a fish bone stuck in her throat; I then realised to my horror, it was my sister! I can recall being frightened for her, for I loved her so much. Thankfully, she was OK, but in that moment, I felt fear that I might lose my sister.

I had happy memories too. It was at that school I also learned that if you want something in life, then go for it.

It was a sunny Friday afternoon. Along with the others in my class, we were told about a race. With our shoes, blazers, hats and satchels laid out along the tennis court, on the whistle, the first to run down the line and get dressed would get to go home early with our parents who were waiting at the end. Wow, I was supercharged that day. I loved my mummy and daddy so much, I gave it my all. My little legs ran like the wind. I really wanted to be at home with them. Winning was my goal that day – if ever a three-year-old could have one. Apart from always being fast on my legs, my subconscious knew from that day that if I wanted something, I could get it through determination. Maybe it was instilled in me then and it is the same for you – if you want something in life, then go for it!

Not so long after that my parents decided, because of my health, to move to Herne Bay in Kent, a coastal town where the air was fresh. We lived in a lovely house in Avenue Road, just around the corner from the sea. We were right opposite a Catholic convent school too and as a Catholic family it was on the cards that we should all go there. I have many more happy memories from my childhood than unhappy ones. I look back and realise that through the different ages and stages of my life, there were challenges and times of hurt. I learned right from wrong and developed a conscience. Through the lessons and the example of my wonderful parents I learned to be kind and show humility, as well as to support others in their need by showing compassion and love.

I grew up to be strong in situations of adversity. But also, indoctrinated with some limiting beliefs such as those old clichés many of my generation remember. I am sure you can recall some of your own!

But despite all that, my parents taught us all to be independent but responsible. To stand true to ourselves, and because of their love we all learned to love.

We had a large extended family and they all flocked to Herne Bay after we settled. I have happy memories of those growing-up years. Religion was a dominating and influencing factor in my life, especially in the formative years. I was an adult before I reconciled some of the challenging aspects of growing up Catholic.

Working in different jobs from a young age, I developed different skills and learned more about the world I was living in. I had some real happy times. But I can also look back and know that there were also challenging situations that I had to get through and deal with, just like all of you. Being mentally abused, made to feel inferior, dealing with grief, work pressure, relationships, miscarriages, births, financial losses, medical intervention, accidents and probably a whole heap more. I could share stories of my pain and survival, but this book is not about that. I got through it.

Depending on the situation I experienced many emotions, such as grief, anger, sadness, bewilderment, shock and fear but then there were many times I experienced emotions of happiness, joy, exhilaration and excitement. That's the way it is in life; we have an experience and just like the game of Snakes and Ladders we can find ourselves feeling up or down. At various stages of my life I have felt broken, hurt, victimised, bullied and mentally abused. I have lacked confidence and had low self-esteem.

Stresses and Traumas

I never recognised them as such but like most, I was a bit blasé as it is all part of life. Engaged at 16, I ended that very challenging relationship two years later. I lost my first baby at 28 weeks at a time when my sisters were both due to give birth to theirs too. After a full labour, not knowing if I had a boy or a girl, to say nothing of pictures, cuddles, footprint, funeral or counselling, I was given a cup of tea and a biscuit and told I could go home in the morning. It was tough!

My second son had to fight for his life at 10 days. Born premature, he weighed only 5lb. With my faith and his fight, he survived. My daughter should have been one of twins, but I lost one at four months. She was born in the back of a car at eight months and it was a miracle she survived.

My children were and still are very precious to me. When my eldest was six, my husband and I divorced. A sad time indeed but things had not been right for a while. I had a real battle, however, doing what I knew to be right; coming from a staunch Catholic family, it came with challenges.

There was once an occasion I felt so low I wanted to block the pain – and although it was never my intention, I almost ended my own life. Love pulled me through, and my now amazing husband, who was a new partner at the time, saved my life. By then I promised myself, no matter how hard life hit me, nothing was going to break me again.

I have been through burglary, mental and emotional abuse, financial struggles relationships, work stress and overwhelm. I share this because I want you to know that although my life has been predominantly a good and happy one, I, like you, do not always know what is around the corner. But I got through in my own way, as you can. My father always used to say 'You do not know what I feel unless you have walked a mile in my shoes.' I have walked some miles, but there are plenty of others that have walked far more.

Following My Dream

I loved working; I had my first job aged 13. When I left school, finding work was very different. If you left a job one day, you were in another the next. From paper rounds and Saturday jobs, to office, retail and farming, I gained experiences in anything and everything. As a young mum I went into sales, then set up my own business in retail and after 10 years embarked on a degree course. I changed direction and went into education. After three degrees I furthered my learning into yoga teaching and therapies. After 17 years in education, in 2010, a fortuitous situation gave me the opportunity to step out. The time was right.

Initially I enjoyed being free to do what I wanted. I continued to teach yoga around the community as, by then after 16 years, I had a following. But barely 10 months had passed, and I soon realised I was not ready to hang up my boots! I had a dream to have my own yoga studio and the perfect place came my way. Life was to take another turn as I was soon to realise another dream! Armed with a broad range of extensive skills from my life's journey, little did I know how important they would be going into the next phase of my life.

> **'The light of awareness always gives rise to new beginnings.'**
>
> *Wallace Huey*
> *Co-founder of Trans4mind Ltd and*
> *author of 'Unfold Your Wings and Watch Life Take Off'*

Caroline's Points to Ponder

1. What are your earliest memories?

2. Are your childhood memories predominantly happy ones?

3. What stresses and traumas have you had?

'Synchronicity is an inexplicable and profoundly meaningful coincidence that stirs the soul and offers a glimpse of one's destiny.'

Phil Cousineau
US author and director of The Hero's Journey

Chapter Three
Synchronicity –
By Not So Strange Coincidence

I am a great believer in synchronicity – things always happen for a reason. Sometimes we might not understand the drive behind an extraordinary happening, but it reveals itself when the time is right.

Back in 1981 when I was in retail, in my one-stop wedding emporium, my husband Terry was a photographer. Before the digital era, films were developed in darkrooms and labs. One day we were told the owner of the labs we used to develop the pictures was dying of cancer. It was a horrible shock, although I did not know him as well as Terry did. I insisted we go and visit him; it seemed the right thing to do.

We went on a sunny Sunday afternoon and took some flowers for his wife. I could see she was pleased to see us even though I had not met her before. We went into the lounge and sat down; he was tucked up on the sofa, clearly a sick man. Terry sat and chatted with him and I with his wife. We were not looking to overstay our welcome, but before leaving, I went over to the sofa, sat down and took the man's hand. Difficult to know what to say in such circumstances. I said I was sorry he was suffering and I thanked him for all the good work he had done.

He held my hand, looked at me and said, 'You are going to do great work and achieve something quite amazing.' I was taken aback – I did not really know what to say! How does someone who does not really know you, get to say those words? Was it a spiritual realisation that, as a dying man, he could sense? I put it to the back of my mind until about a year ago when amazing things were happening with my work. Then his words returned to me. He was right!

My whole life seems to have unfolded in a way that has led me to this journey I want to share with you. For the skills and opportunities I have learned and experienced, and the people I have met on the way, I offer my sincere gratitude. For I need and use all those skills today from youth work, business and education: formal, holistic and spiritual.

> **'Coincidence is the language of the stars.**
> **For something to happen,**
> **so many forces have to be put into action.'**
>
> *Paulo Coelho*
> *Author of 'The Alchemist'*

Before I opened my own yoga studio, I was teaching classes, as always, in the church and community halls of the surrounding area. Prior to going off to teach a class one evening, I received an email from one of my students. 'Have you heard of this?' she asked. I quickly clicked on the link, as I was soon to dash out of the door to go and teach the class. When I arrived, she asked me with enthusiasm if I had received her email. 'Yes,' I replied, 'I did take a look. I have never heard of it and have no idea what it is. But how did you hear about it?' My student said, 'I went upcountry to stay with a friend and she had a visitor from South Africa who told us about it and it sounds amazing. Thought I'd pass it on to you.'

I went home that night and, of all the things I could have done, I was drawn to take another look. What I saw was a picture of David Berceli from the USA along with lots of fascinating information about his Trauma Prevention Exercise training in South Africa. I decided I wanted to go to South Africa to go on the training course and meet David Berceli.

Now here's a thing. At this time, my daughter was living in South Africa. She was coming close to the birth of her first baby. Like any good mum, I was saying to her, 'Don't you worry, we shall be out there for the birth.' But, of course, birth like death, comes when it is ready. We were getting closer and closer to the time but that little voice inside (you know the one I mean) was saying *Don't buy your flight tickets yet.* I am glad I listened, for that little voice was right.

I made a phone call to South Africa that evening and spoke to an English doctor who was organising the course. Before I went to bed that night, I bought two tickets to South Africa. Not only was David Berceli delivering the training around the time of the forthcoming birth, but when the event organiser told me where it was, I said, 'I know that venue. It's only five minutes from where my daughter lives!' *How does that happen?* I booked myself onto the training. To this day I genuinely believe that the Trauma Prevention Exercise training found me.

We arrived in South Africa on the Monday and our beautiful grandson James was born on the Wednesday. On the Friday I was at the already familiar venue together with 99 other people from around the world, to learn a technique called 'Trauma Prevention Exercise'. It was essentially seven key exercises that allowed the body to release held tension from trauma.

The exercises were published in a book David had written from which anyone could easily learn. We were taught these exercises were key for the 'tremoring response*' to happen. Allowing the tremor response is a life-preserving action which discharges adrenalin and cortisol, preventing the body from holding on to dangerously toxic chemicals. On the training, David's sharing of the physiological side of things was insightful. I was struck by the depth of his passion for his work in the rediscovery of what the body can do and what it *should* have been doing all along after every traumatic episode that takes us into 'fight, flight, freeze'. It is this costly inability to let go that leads to the sometimes fatal, physiological breakdown of the body's systems. When we say stress is a silent killer, the very simplified explanation above tells us how.

It was an interesting and fascinating experience. I always say be careful what you wish for. At the end of the three days, without the slightest notion of what it would entail, I stood up in front of 99 other people and declared, 'I am going back to make this happen in the UK.' The rest of

* See glossary at the back for the full meaning.

the world seemed to know about this, but we didn't. I felt strongly enough even then to know that had to change. On my return I set up TRE UK®. My dream yoga centre was ready to go. Terry had worked hard and created a beautiful ambient space. It was literally all I had dreamed of. When we opened, yoga classes started to fill up. I also started to work with case study clients with the TRE. It was a challenge getting people to step into the zone and try something new. My enthusiasm for the work was fuelled by the remarkable healing from the very first person I worked with who started to show me that the body can truly heal itself. I discovered from the start I had something special going on and I knew my life was never going to be the same again. I had a responsibility to share and that was what I was going to do. That promise I made in South Africa? I meant it.

> **'Wisdom is the abstract of the past,
> but beauty is the promise of the future.'**
>
> *Oliver Wendell Holmes Sr
> American physician*

Caroline's Points to Ponder

1. Do you recall any experiences of synchronicity?

2. Have you ever wished for something and it manifested?

3. What was the biggest promise you ever made, and did you see it through?

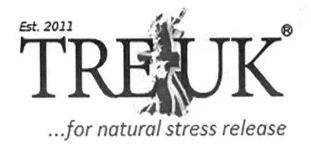

'Believe it can be done.
When you believe something
can be done, really believe,
your mind will find the way to do it.
Believing a solution paves
the way to the solution.'

David J Schwartz
Motivational coach and author of 'The Magic of Thinking Big'

Chapter Four
Square Peg in a Round Hole

When I returned to the UK, I was excited. From the very start I had a unique passion for this new work and yet I still had so much to learn.

I completed the required case studies and was highly praised by my South African mentor. I always dedicate myself to making sure I give everything my best. Being at university, that feeling of not being as clever as all the youngsters (I was 38 when I started my degree studies) was my justification for working hard. I always held the philosophy that hard work pays off. I made notes on all my clients' releasing patterns and I accumulated emails as people asked their questions, shared their joys, frustrations, and challenges, every one of them a rich learning experience, more than any training ever gave me. But I could understand why – it really was experiential. For example, no one could give me the answer to the question as to whether there should be any caution if someone had acid reflux. If you had not worked with that problem, how would you know? The more I saw, the more I learned, and I learned even more by staying in contact with my clients.

Once qualified, I felt proud and excited about moving forward. But that was when things started to change. I asked my mentor the typical question that I now get asked by a lot of people. 'What do I have to do to train to teach others?' I was passionate and wanted to share. I just wanted to know the next steps, when I was ready. In the UK that is what we do. I was told I had to be invited. Now that threw me a bit as I did not know who could invite me! No one knew me!

Anyway, I was put forward and had an online interview with a lady in the USA. She first asked me about myself and I shared my background with her. She said, 'You sound like someone we could do with.' As I was newly qualified, I asked her about the structure of the organisation and who to go to with my questions. She replied, 'Have you seen *The Wizard of Oz*?"

I wanted to know that when I felt ready, what was the next step. OMG, the wind was soon taken out of my sails! It seemed like I had opened a can of worms. In the UK we think and do things very differently from other countries, especially the USA. Our language and expectations are clearly not the same. For whatever reason, my question (and others) seemed to have been taken out of context and I felt very misunderstood. I met resistance. It seemed to me the rules were being made up as they went along. I was not invited to join!

From then on, without wasting my energy on the whys and wherefores, I felt ostracised for my enthusiasm. I had a lot to offer but realised that politics were the order of the day. Politics are not my thing and it was clear I was never going to be welcomed. I just felt blessed that my initial learning was with David, both in South Africa and Germany. There came a point though, (for the second time in my life) where enough was enough! It was a challenging time and I soon realised I was on my own.

I had not done anything to deserve the cold shoulder. Saddened as I was, I just had to hold my head up and do what my heart knew to be right – get on with sharing and helping people move forward from their stress and trauma.

In 2013 I read Professor Gordon Turnbull's book *Trauma: From Lockerbie to 7/7*. In this incredible book, he describes a situation when he was learning from those at the top of their profession. 'They were forceful, highly knowledgeable characters; they did not like to be challenged. I wasn't remotely interested in challenging them, I was interested in learning...'

It took him back to his school days and Miss Roberts' class. He writes, 'I was being penalised for my own curiosity and it didn't feel right. In fact, it made me downright furious. Ultimately, though, any awkwardness or criticism that I experienced with these figures led to *improved* self-insight on my part. I wondered where in medicine could I find a discipline that allowed me to remain a square peg in a round hole – an enthusiast in a world of characters who would inevitably interpret that trait as a challenge?'

When I read his words, I almost cried! That was exactly how I felt. An overwhelming sense of relief came over me. I breathed a big sigh at the realisation that it was not me. That I was OK and had done nothing wrong. I too was hungry to learn, not compete. I was and always have been a team player. I wanted to join this TRE team but, alas, I too was just another square peg in a round hole. Onwards and upwards!

'Life will give you whatever experience is most helpful for the evolution of your consciousness.
How do you know this is the experience you need?
Because this is the experience you are having
at the moment.'

Eckhart Tolle
Spiritual teacher and best-selling author of
'The Power of Now'

Caroline's Points to Ponder

1. Was there a time in your life where you were knocked back?

2. Have you ever read anything that changed your perception about yourself?

3. Have you ever felt you were a square peg in a round hole?

*'When we are no longer able
to change a situation,
we are challenged
to change ourselves.'*

*Viktor Frankl
Neurologist and best-selling author of
'Man's Search for Meaning'*

Part II – A Calling to Initiate Change
Chapter Five
Stress, Trauma and TRE in Context

Imagine you are walking home from work, alone. It's just starting to get dark. You sense, rather than hear, that someone is walking behind you. The hairs on the back of your neck go up: you hold your breath as you listen for footsteps and try to assess the location of the threat. Your muscles tense, and your heart pounds as adrenalin and other chemicals cascade through your body. You might notice you have started sweating and your tummy suddenly feels full of butterflies as you quicken your pace. If you feel totally trapped and can see no escape from whatever is behind you, you may even 'freeze' in panic, feeling completely overwhelmed and helpless.

Fortunately, you make it home unharmed. As you unlock the door, you realise your hands are shaking so much you can hardly get the key in the lock. Your legs feel wobbly and your teeth are chattering. 'Don't be silly,' you tell yourself. 'There was no one there ... just your imagination. Pull yourself together!' As you head for a cup of tea, or reach for a glass of something stronger, you tell yourself to stop trembling. After all, it's embarrassing, unnatural and a bit weak and feeble, isn't it? Well, no, not really.

The effects of trauma

Unreleased tension stemming from traumatic situations can contribute to many maladies and conditions, including anxiety disorders, addictions, insomnia, depression, gastrointestinal problems, fibromyalgia, high blood pressure, migraines, fatigue, and unexplained aches and pains. When the human body is under perpetual physiological duress caused by fight, flight or freeze, there are serious consequences and it is likely **all** disease is worsened by it. The resources that would otherwise be employed maintaining the health of the body's systems, including the immune system, are diverted to maintaining the state of physiological panic. Over time, this impairs the healthy functioning of the body in multiple ways.

It's important to note here, although trauma *contributes* to illness, once the illness has become 'somatised'* that is, present in the body on a physical level, it must be treated appropriately across the board.

Trauma-related symptoms affect not only the sufferer, but often have a devastating impact on family, friends and work colleagues, too. People who are constantly on edge, irritable or angry are not good at fostering positive relationships, particularly if they tend to overreact and fly off the handle at the slightest provocation. Trauma survivors can be hard to love. Through no fault of their own, they may appear disconnected, distracted and reluctant to share their feelings. This can alienate their nearest and dearest who, while remaining sympathetic, often feel they simply can't cope.

Symptoms are also notoriously hard to pin down. They don't necessarily appear immediately following an incident and may take months or even years to surface, and then only gradually. As a result, people often suffer for years from physical and psychological complaints but are not sure why. They try all kinds of treatments and therapies, some of which may provide some relief but, because they do not address the underlying issues, are generally doomed to failure.

* *See glossary at the back for the full meaning.*

Life is traumatic

Most people have heard of Post-Traumatic Stress Disorder, (PTSD*) but usually assume it relates only to military personnel, refugees, or people who have survived major disasters such as wars, terrorist attacks, earthquakes, fire, flooding, and so on. Yet each one of us can be affected by post-traumatic stress.

Accidents of any kind have a huge impact not only on the victim, but also witnesses, onlookers, medical teams, family, and friends. Physical and mental abuse scar mind and body, and serious illness and surgery can also leave their marks long after the event and the apparent recovery period. You can perhaps have been traumatised by any number of ordinary and extraordinary experiences. Starting or leaving school, relationship problems, issues at work, unemployment, bereavement, giving birth, an abusive and or neglectful childhood, poverty, chronic illness (your own or your loved ones'), disability, persistent worry …the list is endless. Although some of these incidents may not register as traumatic at the time, and you may well have forgotten them, your body remembers.

When you recognise that even thinking stressful thoughts can cause a rush of fight, flight or freeze hormones and chemicals, it's easy to see that the daily challenges you face have the potential to leave you tense, angry and on edge. A disagreement with the boss, rushing to get the kids from school, or a row with a partner can all temporarily disturb the balance of your nervous system. When your body is operating optimally, it will naturally reset itself after a deranging event. Problems arise when it doesn't and develops instead a maladaptive stress response, as can happen after a significant traumatic event or years of minor ones that simply add up.

However, although your mind-body system perceives mildly stressful situations like these as threats, you are unlikely to respond with physical action. Even if you feel like punching your boss, screaming at the kids or attacking the person who cut in front of your car, hopefully, reason intervenes and you restrain yourself. If you were any kind of mammal other than human, in your natural state, you would either fight or run

* *See glossary at the back for the full meaning.*

when threatened. Afterwards, you'd have a good shake to release any energy left over from the event, thereby resetting your nervous system. But for us humans, our body's ideal option of either fight or flight is often neither enacted nor resolved with a good natural shake. The initial surge of emotional energy remains, leaving us awash with a raft of biochemicals designed to be burned off by energetic action. Worse still, our third biological option of temporarily freezing until the danger has passed can set in long term, fossilizing us in a debilitating frozen state of physiological panic for hours, weeks or even years.

Containing this powerful tension within you takes a great deal of energy – one reason why people suffering from post-traumatic stress are often easily fatigued.

The healing power within

The answer, as it often does, lies within you. Deep in your core is a set of powerful muscles called the psoas* group; we shall explore these more in the next chapter. Each time you experience a fearful event, notice how you instinctively contract to protect yourself. This has the effect of pulling your body forward into a curved position to safeguard the areas that are most vulnerable – your face, heart, lungs and abdomen.

This response is instinctive and universal. All people, faced with a threatening situation, will experience the same kind of muscular contraction. This fact came to the attention of aforementioned David Berceli, a somatic therapist. During his experiences in Middle Eastern war zones, he noticed that soldiers all made the same involuntary movement to protect their bodies when explosions occurred. As a body therapist, Berceli recognised this movement was created by specific muscle patterns, and if repeated, could lead to a build-up of excess tension. He questioned whether if in releasing this chronic muscle tension, he might also be able to help people release trauma-related stress from the system. He also observed that tremoring during or after stressful or dangerous situations was innate to people of many cultures.

* *See glossary at the back for the full meaning.*

Putting the above findings together, he realised the human body is innately capable of activating this involuntary 'shaking' mechanism to release tension and restore balance to the system.

Berceli went on to develop a system of seven exercises to activate this instinctive shaking mechanism in the body by stressing the psoas muscles to induce tremoring. As he hoped, after tremoring sessions his clients reported not only a feeling of physical relaxation but also a sense of emotional release and well-being.

While Trauma Prevention Exercises significantly help release trapped energy and prevent future disease, they won't on their own heal, for example, a chronic viral or inflammatory disease, even if these conditions are facilitated by trauma-induced failures in a person's immunity. Diet and other lifestyle considerations play an important part if TRE is to have the best possible chance of realising its essential power.

'O Lord heal me, for my bones are shaking with terror'

Psalm 6:2

Caroline's Points to Ponder

1. Do you recall a time when you had butterflies?

2. Did you know that all your stressful or traumatic experiences impacted your health?

3. Have you ever considered the idea that your body can heal itself?

*'Fear is lodged in our bodies.
It vibrates in the nervous system
and is easily evoked.
Although fear is often a subtle
experience, we attempt to control
this unpleasant feeling of anxiety
by adding more muscular tension,
resulting in layer upon
layer of rigidity.'*

Liz Koch
*Somatic Educator, creator of Core Awareness, and
best-selling author of 'The Psoas Book'*

Chapter Six
The Healing Power Within, the Inertia of Today's Solutions and Why They Don't Work!

The Psoas – Our Best Kept Secret

To say the psoas muscle is the best kept secret is an understatement. Do you know where your psoas muscle is? Why would you know? The majority of people, when asked, draw a complete blank. Even some in the medical profession are never sure. No surprise though. Let me explain.

The psoas is not easily accessed; you cannot go and get it massaged. It is in your back body, under your diaphragm and runs down behind your organs, like a protective cloak. Apart from holding your upper body to your lower body and allowing flexion of your legs, it also supports your posture.

Most importantly it is your fight/flight centre, where you hold emotions and fears and because it is attached to the diaphragm, not surprisingly, it can impact your breathing.

The psoas muscle is the primary muscle that contracts to protect your centre of gravity in a fearful situation. During danger, there is a reaction causing an intricate interaction of biological, neurological, and nervous systems. This interaction causes the muscle to contract to protect you from harm or possible death. The psoas is the primary muscle that activates your flight/flight and freeze response and reacts instinctually to a perceived danger, which is not under your conscious control. This core muscle rolls your body into a foetal position, protecting your vital organs and the soft vulnerable parts of your body as well as providing resiliency to the spine to help your body sustain a blow or fall.

Your emotions are your responses to events of stress and fear, but also serve you after the event has passed to protect you from further, similar experiences that could cause you more physical or psychological harm. However, such feelings are stored in your brain and body.

Both the brain and the psoas muscle are linked to your nervous system, which regulates your future responses to stress; this way, past but unreleased experiences lead you to react in a way that is meant to protect you. Which is often why you may react to events in a disproportionate manner by 'overreacting,' as stressed people often do.

Research has now caught up with the knowledge that your life experiences are stored in your body's muscle memory and you continue, unknowingly, to hold tension and trauma until you physically release what is held and undischarged.

Your ability to cope with and recover from stress and trauma is often compromised because you often simply do not have sufficient time to process what has happened to you, particularly nowadays when the pace of life is so rapid. Today, people are routinely discharged the next day after surgery, when the body is still in a state of shock. Nursing or convalescent homes, which allowed people time to recover from operations or illness, have virtually vanished. A period of mourning used to follow bereavement, when not very much was expected of the bereaved. Now we are expected to get back to work as soon as possible after the burial or cremation and somehow expected to fit our grieving in between everything else we must do.

Numerous symptoms start off being niggling but then seem to take over, until physically, mentally and emotionally you can hit rock bottom. You suffer from back pain, neck or shoulder pain, Irritable Bowel Syndrome, headaches, insomnia, tearfulness, anger, anxiety, depression. At worst, a stroke, heart attack, cancer, or even suicide.

It is for this reason we have to manage stress – we have to take responsibility, because stress is not a silent killer, we are just letting it kill us by not dealing with it.

'But I don't have any stress!' is something I hear all too often. Not now maybe, but your body is still sitting with the impact from past stress or past trauma, much of which you don't remember, especially from childhood. You may even have taken on stress in your mother's womb. Being in denial is costly. However, for those that do notice the ailments that start to manifest, there are three key options:

1. Talk therapy

2. Medication

3. Self-medication

What are they and why don't they work?

Talk Therapy

Traditional talking therapies such as Cognitive Behaviour Therapy (CBT)* can help people deal with post-traumatic stress, but they don't suit everyone. Some people find their painful experiences impossible to put into words, or perhaps their memories of the event are too fragmented or confused to express verbally. Others may be reluctant to 'make a fuss'. As a nation, we are rather proud of our 'stiff upper lip'. Bottling up emotions and fears rather than expressing them is seen as a virtue by many. Those who **do** let go of their emotions, particularly if they are leaders, run the risk of being dubbed weak or overemotional.

Talking to family, friends and colleagues does not necessarily help either. If the person keeps repeating their story and going over and over the same old ground as trauma survivors tend to, their listeners are likely to lose patience with them. Remarks such as 'Just get over it!' or 'It's time you moved on,' can cause the person to withdraw or even try to belittle their own experience.

* *See glossary at the back for the full meaning.*

From working in schools, it is clear young people certainly do not want to talk or open up. They then further suppress their feelings, creating more tension.

Medication

Going to the doctor is what we have been conditioned to do. Aches, pains, feeling out of sorts; on every level, the doctor can fix us. However, they have no magic wand. They can give medication for the pains, the anxiety, the depression, the lack of sleep or anything else. Have you read the insert of cautions and side effects of some of these medications? Crikey, they scare the life out of me! The problem with medication is that it is a bit like a sticky plaster, covering over the wound but not addressing the cause of the wound itself.

While appropriate medication has its place, and can be very helpful in some cases, many people are reluctant to take drugs, particularly on a long-term basis, because of side effects and dependence issues. It is certainly not ideal to put a young person on antidepressants either.

Self-medication

Well, this is certainly the option we may get most comfort from because we choose what makes us feel temporarily better. From drugs and alcohol to gambling or excessive exercise, from eating to getting hooked into social media. There are many Obsessive-Compulsive Disorder (OCD)* behaviours that in the short-term mask our symptoms and block our feelings, especially in suppressing blocked anger, finding it difficult to concentrate or absorb new information. It is therefore not uncommon to turn our repressed anger and frustration on ourselves, via self-harming, over-eating, or abusing alcohol or drugs.

Whatever option you choose, none of them are healthy, and before you know it, you have an addiction to deal with.

* *See glossary at the back for the full meaning.*

So, what else?

Take your pick. A lot depends on your disposable income. Massage to try ease the back pain and the tension in your body's muscles. Tapping or reiki to try shift energy blocks. Holidays or retreats to get away from it all. Weekly classes of yoga, tai chi, mindfulness, meditation to be in the moment. Hypnotism, frog poison in the Amazon. Goodness, how long have you got and, more to the point, how much money have you got?!

I always remember running a Workshop for a group of women. Between them they had spent a grand total of £170k - **yes indeed, not a misprint!** - spent £170k on trying to get someone or something to fix them!

They sat in front of me with hope in their eyes. They left with hope in their hearts. For there was that one thing they had not tried – allowing their body to heal itself!

So how can you get to grips with unreleased tension, stress and trauma? What if there were an easy way to get rid of blocked energy gently and safely without having to resort to pills, alcohol, or outside intervention?

Animal wisdom

When it comes to dealing with trauma, we can learn a lot from the animal kingdom. Unlike us, wild animals (when not held captive) get rid of any blocked energy very efficiently. As trauma expert Peter A. Levine observed in *Waking the Tiger: Healing Trauma*, a gazelle that survives an attack by a predator, such as a lion, will shake and shiver for a while once the danger has passed, then return to peaceful grazing with the rest of the herd. This protective mechanism has obvious benefits. As Levine says, 'It is difficult to imagine how individual wild animals (or their entire species, for that matter) would have ever survived if they routinely developed the sorts of debilitating symptoms that many humans do.'

While we are not at risk of being pursued by lions in the course of our daily life, we are all exposed to various other forms of trauma from birth right through to adulthood.

The somatic response to over-excitement or fear is to tremor. Studies on animal behaviour show how tremoring protects them from psychological and physical damage after a frightening experience. Well here's the thing – we are all animals. As David Attenborough once said, 'We are animals in clothing.' Humans too have this built-in mechanism to tremor. To release from the body in this way is necessary to return homeostasis (balance) to the body and mind after shock or stress. Animals and humans cannot prevent trauma, nor can trauma be prevented, but whatever you go through in your life, the body has the mechanism to release it.

Have you ever had the experience of being unable to control overwhelming emotions? Maybe your lips quivered, your legs or hands shook involuntarily. This tremor sensation is the body's most organic method of releasing tension that has become charged within the system. Such tremoring or shaking has been and still is seen as a pathological weakness. As a consequence, we freeze or suppress the response – and then we are on that downwards spiral.

You can empower yourself like so many others to return to homeostasis by reconnecting with what nature gave you – just like animals! In our empowering and healing programme, you start immediately to heal from the past and begin to build resilience.

Tremors come from the centre of gravity of the body (S3) which is protected by the psoas muscles. When neurogenic tremors are evoked at this powerful centre, where the protective pattern of contraction was created, the vibrations reverberate through the entire body travelling along the spine, releasing tension from stress and trauma from both body and mind. It is precisely this tremor mechanism that needs to be reactivated, particularly after a traumatic event. This response stimulates the parasympathetic nervous system, discharging tension in the muscles, reducing high biochemical levels and restoring healthy balance. This combination of effects helps to turn off the organism's emergency protective response – fight or flight – restoring it to normal calm functioning.

'Psychogenic tremors in humans, much the same as the instinctual tremors in animals, is the natural response of a shocked or disrupted nervous system attempting to restore the Neuro-physiologic homeostasis of the body.'

Feldman, 2004; Van der Kolk and Van der Hart, 1991

Caroline's Points to Ponder

1. Did you know where your psoas is?

2. What 'niggles' have you noticed in your body?

3. Do you recall your body ever shaking following a difficult or frightening situation?

'Every experience in your life is being orchestrated to teach you something you need to know to move you forward.'

Brian Tracy
Public speaker and best-selling author of
'The Psychology of Achievement'

Chapter Seven
On Becoming an Expert and a Special Connection

Since 2012 I have been working with clients from all walks of life. Inevitably my programme has evolved to incorporate the many experiences and knowledge gleaned over the years. I know my 'stuff'. I am somewhat of an expert in a unique field of work.

So how did I get to earn this title? On return from South Africa where I learned the TRE method from David, I opened my yoga centre, set up TRE UK® and created a website to start sharing what I knew. I worked through case studies first with four individuals and then one small group. Beyond my qualification, I began to have a flow of people seeking to learn as word was slowly spreading. Being a new concept of healing requiring a complete mindset shift, I was under no illusion that it was going to be an overnight sensation.

I learned from every 'body' I supported with their release. I was observing remarkable release patterns and receiving more and more feedback as everyone shared their story on how they were healing and slowly transforming their life.

The Universe works in strange ways

In 2013 I received a call from Heidi, asking if she could come to my yoga classes. She had moved nearby to temporarily nurse her father dying of cancer. He lived in one of the flats on the seafront just along the way from my yoga studio. When she came to the classes, she loved the experience.

She often stayed behind and we would chat over coffee. We really seemed to connect. She attended classes quite frequently over a three-week period before her father died. She was then, as one might expect, grief-stricken. This was when I said to her, 'Heidi, it's time to do my practice.' By the time she had finished a six-session course with me, she couldn't believe how quickly she had overcome her grief and was able to function on all levels with calm and peace.

She continued with yoga while she was sorting out her father's affairs in Dover before moving back home. She stayed in touch and I was glad to have connected with her. I didn't realise how much until she called me up one day and asked if I would work with a friend of hers – Katherine – who was going through an acrimonious divorce. She told me Katherine was incredibly angry and having tried everything, wanted to connect with me to find out more about the TRE. I said, 'Of course, I will be happy to work with her!'

'Great,' she replied. 'Oh, and by the way, she is a journalist with the *Daily Mail* and has been given permission to write about it.' OMG, I did not see that coming! I thought to myself, 'This could either be the shortest career in history or it may go somewhere.' But she wrote a very positive article. I was quite blown away. I had 4,000 hits on my website that day, but more significantly, a full mailbox, from Land's End to John O'Groats.

Each email was from someone suffering silently, having tried everything to no avail to heal their trauma. They were now looking for hope from me as they had read the story in the *Daily Mail* of the profound benefits my client wrote about. They too wanted to heal from all their physical, mental or emotional problems.

The Universe had been listening. Daunting as it was, I had to plan. I felt proud to give TRE the first big UK news splash, but it was now time to work out what to do.

I had two websites set up, one for the yoga centre and one for TRE UK®. I decided that to start reaching out, I would plan a mini tour. An Events page was added to the website to include a map of the UK that would highlight the towns and cities I would be visiting.

One coincidence after another!

I had a private client in Bromley call to make a booking for me to visit her house so she could learn the practice. I arranged it for the Wednesday of the same week that I was in London on the Friday.

On Tuesday evening, I received a text message which I picked up after teaching my yoga class. It was quite a desperate plea for help. The message indicated that the sender was very scared as she was shaking like mad and could not stop. I messaged back asking her what she had done. She replied that she had done TRE from a YouTube video; I called her immediately. She was in turmoil. She watched someone on YouTube delivering seven exercises, and apparently when nothing happened the clip just finished with, 'Well there it is'. She lay on her sofa, and then all of a sudden started to shake, and couldn't stop. Furthermore, her young son walked into the room and was frightened to see his mother this way. I asked her if she had been through trauma. She said her whole life had been traumatic. I said, 'You have let the tiger out of the cage and do not know how to rein him back in.' I also informed her that it was an immensely powerful practice and she needed to learn properly.

I asked where she lived. Now of all the places in England, and guess what was her reply was? Bromley! 'Goodness,' I said, 'this is your lucky day as I am in Bromley tomorrow!' I arranged to visit her at lunchtime. As luck would have it, she was no more than a 10-minute drive away and when I met her, we had a long chat. The second stroke of luck for her too was that I was in London on the Friday, so needless to say, she booked on to the event. So, we met again. She left that day happy that she was able to have the experience that she did.

Getting the show on the road

Back to my mini tour. I had mapped out and created a schedule that would cover 1,400 miles. I would deliver five events from Somerset to Manchester and locations in between. For various reasons I had to go by myself. Venues and B & Bs all booked, I packed up the car and set off. My planned programme included split presentations and two practical sessions, for the four-hour event. My resources were limited but everyone seemed happy with the essentials they received. Despite having worked with quite a lot of people and seeing bodies do extraordinary things, I was under no illusion this week was going to be a steep learning curve.

I then went on to Northampton to work with a lady who had Parkinson's. I guess with my growing faith that the body will never take one to a place of harm, so when asked if the TRE would help with her condition, I had no reason to think that it wouldn't. When I arrived at the lady's flat, I thought to myself, 'OMG she is trembling with Parkinson's; how will I know the difference?' Well, I did and after the session she felt calm and happy and knew something had changed. We chatted for a while and before I left, she said, 'Goodness, look at me! I have been standing here for over 45 minutes and without medication, I am not shaking!' I was so happy for her. So, I realised that TRE is good for Parkinson's! We kept in touch and yes, she continued with the practice. What she also shared is that she had a new confidence, to speak out and contribute in meetings and be in the company of others. How wonderful.

Each Workshop had between 6 and 12 participants and I have such special memories of all the individuals I met and what I learned from them. The experience was incredible as each and every one taught me more about releasing bodies, inner fears and the internal battle of wanting to heal but not wanting to experience the potential reactions that could come up. These observations continued to influence my message.

My presentation was initially based around what I had learned in South Africa which was very much trauma focused. After each event I found myself 'tweaking' my message, slowly, slowly over time to become a little more uplifting. I was daring to be different.

Having got through the week, I started to plan more events always on the weekend as I had yoga classes to teach in the week. I was also teaching a couple of groups with the TRE too. Life was busy and I realised that this was how it was going to be. I had some important work to do.

My journey had well and truly started – every day I continued to learn something new and shudder when I think of the responsibility I took on. I was meeting people with all sorts of physical, mental and emotional problems. Doing my own practice, I felt strong and resilient to be able to deal with them and give advice and guidance from experience. Intuition played a big part, particularly as I was not getting help or support from anywhere else. I recognised that no one had been able to answer the questions I had asked in the past because they hadn't encountered the experience themselves! Experience was key; the practice was and always will be, in my view, 'experiential'.

No two people are the same; every one of us is different. We have all evolved from our own unique past. That is what has shaped us and who we are as individuals. So therefore, the releasing of the negative aspects of that past is going to be different for everyone. To this day, that is what I love, always seeing something different. Amazing sharings and stories about the weird and wonderful releasing experiences would drop daily into my email box, and they still do.

A Special Connection

One of those first events was at Horton Cross, Somerset. A good group came together. At the end one lady said to me, 'I would love you to meet Professor Gordon Turnbull'. She was a client of his, so gave me his number. I, of course, had not heard of him and didn't do anything with it at first. But then another lady I worked with on my return to Somerset also spoke to me about him. Then a third person called hoping I could work with her ex-military husband, and when I asked her how she found out about my work, she said, 'Professor Turnbull'. That was it – where was that number?!

I dialled and was quite taken aback when he answered the phone. To this day, his words from that first conversation still resonate with me. 'We now know we have to get it [trauma] out of the body, talking just doesn't do it'. We chatted for ages and I felt a real warm connection with him. I said that I hoped one day we would meet, and we certainly did, but not until 2014.

It was in this conversation that he asked me if I knew Mandy Bostwick. I didn't; however, he spoke well of her and suggested I contact her. She had done her degree in Trauma Psychology under his tutelage at Chester University. So I called her and we clicked straight away. We chatted for ages and a new friendship was beginning. When I went to Chester to deliver a planned event, Mandy insisted we stayed with her. I was excited to meet her.

A couple of years later, Mandy observed a Chester Workshop (moving on from events). After the first session when all were resting out, she had tears in her eyes. She could not believe what she was seeing. She said, 'I have been writing about energy for years, but I have never seen anything like this.'

Mandy specialises in working with veterans' trauma and veterans in prisons. Sharing time with her, I came to learn more and more about trauma and the impact on the body. It felt great to know that whatever came up for my clients in releasing, I would have the expertise of a trauma specialist to connect with and discuss issues. It was a reassuring safeguard for my clients and enhanced my own knowledge and brought anything I read in a book to life. Equally, Mandy was fascinated to hear my stories about different ways the body would let go and truly heal.

In August 2014, Professor Turnbull offered me the chance to work with some of his clients in the Capio Nightingale Hospital in London. I felt it was an extreme honour. I will say little about the experience out of respect for the clients I worked with. However, what I experienced in this work was the privilege of dealing with one of the most highly traumatised clients I have ever seen. To see week on week the shift from total fear such as I have never witnessed, to some nine weeks later, being able to have a rational conversation and play the guitar was just amazing! The client's father shared with me on one occasion that of all the treatments the client received in over the three months, what I taught had made the most profound impact. He attended a Workshop himself and like all others that discover the power of their own body, was blown away.

In December of that year, I met Gordon for the first time at the hospital and we had a Christmas lunch. Although we had spoken on the phone, meeting him was special. We connected so well and did not stop talking, so much so I had to dash for my train back to Kent as I had to teach in the evening. He signed my copy of his book too, which I shall always treasure. He further invited me to be a guest speaker at the Swindon Trauma Conference which I attended for two years running.

I feel blessed for the challenges that I have been presented with, and those whom have trusted and allowed me to support them: the professionals, veterans, amputees, stroke victims, abused, teenagers, elderly and those with chronic illness, cancer, injuries and Parkinson's. With the thousands of bodies I have seen release, I think it is fair to say I have become an expert!

'Remember that experience creates internalisation.
Doing things repeatedly leads to internalisation,
which produces a quality of understanding that is
generally vastly superior to intellectualised learning.'

Ray Dalio
American philanthropist

Caroline's Points to Ponder

1. Can you recall coincidences in your life?

2. Have you ever met someone who profoundly influenced your life?

3. What has been your most life-changing experience?

*'To improve is to change;
to be perfect is to change often.'*

*Sir Winston Churchill
British Prime Minster and author*

Chapter Eight
Time for Change –
The Total Release Experience® and a New Plan of Action!

I t was in the early days with my new work that I soon began to recognise the resistance that is typically British – the avoidance of talking about their stress, let alone trauma. It became obvious to me if I was going to share what I knew, there had to be some changes. We really are the 'stiff upper lip' brigade, aren't we! No matter what we go through, our philosophy is 'pick ourselves up, dust ourselves off, and start over again'. I can put my own hand up and say many a time that was me!

From a business perspective, towards the end of 2013 it dawned on me that 'Trauma Prevention Exercise' just wasn't working. There was something about the 'trauma' aspect that was not resonating with me or indeed potential clients. Acknowledging stress is a struggle for most, even today, never mind trauma. So many are also in denial. You cannot prevent trauma either if it's going to happen. Being in the wrong place at the wrong time or being in an environment where you are trapped, especially as a child, you have to get through and survive the best you can. The other thing I worked out too was that releasing was by no means reliant on any exercises.

Same, same but different

Time for a change of name that would respect the TRE that David had set up but make it more appealing for the UK. I sat round the table with three friends who had done the practice with me and we brainstormed ideas. I had a light bulb moment and came up with the Total Release Experience®. I felt excited that it would make sharing the TRE more palatable.

I loved the name then and I still do, for it encompasses our whole message that has evolved over time. I had a new logo designed as well as created support resources. I was excited with the changes.

Daniel enters the lion's den!

It is totally relevant here to bring Daniel into the equation. Daniel is my eldest son. He was living in Germany in 2011, married, with three beautiful children. When he came for a visit, he willingly became my guinea pig. He was, as he will tell you now, fascinated and felt good with it. He has a story to tell, which we shall come to later, but he took a real interest in what I was doing and started to work remotely with me as he could sense I was getting submerged with administration as my client base was growing. With his MBA, his skills far superseded mine when it came to systems and structures!

In 2015 he trained to become a practitioner and in 2017 moved back to the UK following his divorce. He was passionate about the work and joined me in building the foundations for the business that was destined to grow from what had been my vision in 2011.

Joined-up thinking

It was great having Daniel on board, especially as by 2014 any connections with the organisation I trained with were over. Not via my choosing, I add, but that is life. Not meant to be and I soon understood why.

Daniel and I are very much aligned in our thinking. He was keen to shadow me in all my work so he too could understand from experience too. He had a head start as I had much to share with him. Although his intention in supporting me was that I would also enjoy a little more freedom, that never really happened! Before long we were both working hard to create, build and evolve in order to share what we know. I ask at times – did he know what he was getting into when he stepped into my world!

Daniel had some great ideas and after every Workshop listening to what I was sharing, he would create ideas. He started with the name, Total Release Experience®, giving it more clarity:

Total: Works on all six essential areas of well-being
Physical, Occupational, Spiritual, Emotional, Social, Intellectual

Release: From yesterday's stress and trauma.

Experience: Build resilience for tomorrow's stress and tomorrow's trauma.

I shall come back to these aspects again.

Furthermore, unless you have that amazing crystal ball then you don't know what is around the corner either. You might find yourself in a situation triggered by a word or an action without even seeing it coming. All those life events that can happen which you may get caught up in. Situations over which you have no control, can change your physical, mental or emotional well-being in a flash. That is why building resilience is so important.

Resilience is having the ability to recover from tough and challenging situations. You, like so many others, may think you are resilient but there is one thing you have overlooked – your body remembers it all.

The more I learned, the more I wanted everyone to hear my message. 'Look, everyone, this is important. You can all heal yourself; you do not have to live with the symptoms of stress anymore.' Many times, it fell (and sadly still does) on deaf ears.

The three reasons people do not connect is because they;

- are scared: it is the fear of the unknown.
- want someone else to make them better.
- do not know enough.

This is still true in 2020 which is why not a week, or a month, goes by when we constantly review the words we share and the practice we teach. Everything now is so different and far removed from what I first learned.

Initially my message was reiterating what I originally learned, trauma and how bad that made us feel. Quite gloomy. It took one lady from Chester to really bring this home – she told me to make my message more uplifting. Well, one thing I do well is listen. Every time someone makes a comment or suggestion, I am not afraid to change.

I believe as a business we should never stand still, we have to keep evolving to ensure the customer experience is always the best it can be. Our message, practice and resources have constantly gone through change. Many clients have been to our Workshops repeatedly over the years, giving their support and positive feedback on the changes we make. I am ever grateful to Daniel for bringing a fresh look – we are a great team!

We now have a language that is shared and understood by all we connect with. From doctors and psychologists to teachers, teenagers, the service sector, the military, prison inmates and individuals from all walks of life.

Our teaching delivers a clear, simple intriguing message:

- This is why you need to release
- This is how you release
- These are the consequences if ignored

Our clients learn three key words to support them on their healing journey:

Diamonds – Buckets – Roller Coasters

**'Learning is experience.
Everything else is just information.'**

*Albert Einstein
Theoretical physicist*

Caroline's Points to Ponder

1. On a scale of 1 (low) to 5 (high), rate the six areas of your well-being.

2. On a scale of 1 to 5, how resilient are you?

3. Which one fits you regarding an unknown healthcare experience?

    a.   Scared – fear of the unknown

    b.   Let someone else do it for me

    c.   Need to know more

*'No Pressure
No Diamond
No Struggle
No Strength.'*

Anon

Chapter Nine
Diamonds, Buckets and the Downward Spiral – Reframing Stress!

Many a time, and I am sure I am not alone, I have sat in anticipation at a workshop, university lecture, conference, or talk, notebook at the ready to write down every word the speaker delivers. Then comes that point and depending on the speaker, I completely switch off. I am sure you have done the same. Why? Because the language is either jargon or complicated – scientific babble that might sound clever but does not make sense. It may do for some, but not me. I like to keep it simple.

When teaching business in schools, I made it my policy to teach students to understand from the base level and build on the idea. I came from a background of experience, not a textbook. It worked for me and my students. We were a successful department and students achieved great results. I have held that philosophy with language for years – why would I change now?

In our teachings we want clients to remember three things – DIAMONDS and BUCKETS are the first two. Let me explain.

DIAMONDS

Diamonds are used in various well-being scenarios, and why not? We know that Diamonds are bright, beautiful, special, and unique.

When we talk of Diamonds, we are not talking about what we wear on our fingers or around our neck; I am not a diamond girl myself. We believe that a little Diamond is formed inside every newborn baby. Like real diamonds before they are formed, they are black, and it takes pressure to bring out the shine. Healthy babies born into loving caring hands will inevitably begin to have that gentle pressure placed on them, to smile, to sit, to feed, to crawl and so on. Encouragement continues through the years with opportunities that help them to grow and in so doing, the Diamond comes out and shines.

Why then is not everyone shining, being the best they can be? Because life has dealt them some tough cards. Maybe that resonates with you. Some babies are not so fortunate. They may have been born via medical intervention or into unloving hands, and suffered abuse, neglect or abandonment. A baby may have a great start in life but then in childhood years, trauma has hit them. Stress overwhelm or trauma can impact a life at any age or stage.

Many clients have shared their story of trauma and tragedy from an early age. For some it seems to have followed them throughout their life. One special lady – I shall call her Rosalind – is a real testimony of courage. The reason she wanted to share parts of her story was because she was frightened by the magnitude of what she wanted to heal from. She needed reassurance from me that she was not a hopeless case.

> *I really appreciate your compassion as, yes, there has been an inordinate number of big traumas in my life from an early age. It began with a major road accident when I was two when my 28-year-old mum lost her leg and unborn child. I had 40 stitches in my face. I was bullied throughout childhood because of my scar. When I was eleven and he was eight, one of my brothers fell over a 70ft cliff (witnessed by our four-year old brother). Miraculously, he survived with minor injuries, reporting that just before he hit the rocks he felt a 'giant hand' lift him up. When asked by a passer-by where he'd come from, he pointed skyward and said, "Up there." He was in all the newspapers.*

Because of her artificial leg, Mum was unable to walk down the cliff path to be with her son. A year or so later, Mum developed breast cancer which led to many disfiguring operations before her premature death when I was 15. From then on, Dad would be a self-employed, lone parent to me and my three younger brothers. Five years later, the same brother who witnessed the cliff fall saw our father take a disabling fall from his window cleaning ladder. Miraculously, a subsequent fall clicked his ankle back into place and he was able to walk again. He would go on to have a debilitating stroke during a vicious attack, witnessed by both me and my three-year old daughter. My youngest daughter, also present at the time, was two months old. A few years after that, Dad had another stroke followed by a coma, before he was finally released into death.

The above details are really the tip of the iceberg and there were several other big traumas. As a family, there is, and always has been, a lot of love between us all and I think this may be what keeps us sane and generally optimistic. As I mentioned to you, I now have a neurological illness. And the patterns of trauma have inevitably resurfaced in the next generation.

For my beloved daughters, it's been in the shape of traumatic surgery, medical negligence injuries, a house fire, a car crash, chronic illness, disability and what we now recognise as PTSD. There was yet another serious fall where, once again, a 'giant hand' came to the rescue. Someone is clearly taking care of us amid the pain and catastrophe. Fortunately, my daughters and I are committed to somehow 'clearing up the mess,' both as soul sisters and blood relatives. When health allows, we continue to research and use a variety of healing modalities. We practise mindfulness as a way of life.

When I came upon Peter Levine's work, it was like finding a key to a locked door. Over the years I've been blessed with synchronicities, much like your story about going to South Africa for the birth of your grandchild and doing your TRE training. I've found many great healers where, no matter how few of them exist in a particular discipline in the UK, there is always one local enough to me that I can get to. Another example of a power greater than myself at work, I assume. The Total Release Experience® is a godsend to me.

When I first read this, I was stunned by the life cards she and her family had been dealt. No wonder her battle in life has been to survive and thrive in the best way possible, but unable to reach full potential and shine her Diamond.

BUCKETS

Back in the '70s psychologists used the phrase 'stress buckets'. We are familiar with the term; we use the term to deliver a very clear message in our education.

Let's take a step back now to put it into context. Remember the psoas muscle from Chapter Six? I want you now to think of it as a container. In fact, think of it as your **Stress Bucket**. From the day you were born, your BUCKET has been filling. It has filled with your HISTORY. We all have HISTORY. You may not remember it all. Your HISTORY includes all the:

Hurt you have ever endured – physically, mentally and emotionally.

Injuries, accidents and operations or anything else inflicted on your body.

Stress – all you can ever remember and a lot you don't.

Trauma – whatever experiences you have had.

Overwhelm – those times in life when you have had a deluge of demands placed upon you and just don't know which way to turn.

Rejection – being abandoned, snubbed, ignored or shunned by loved ones, family, friends, work colleagues or anyone else.

Youth – all those things you may have regrettably done in your teenage years.

So, you can imagine the more HISTORY you go through, the more your BUCKET fills. The fuller it gets, the more your Diamond loses its shine. Simple but clear!

Take a moment to jot down in your notebook incidents from your life that fit into each category.

Let's come back to Rosalind's story:

It was some years later when she attended another Workshop and she told me one of her brothers had taken his own life. Though a man of high standing and one whom she had tried to encourage on numerous occasions to attend a Workshop with her, he never did. With an overfull BUCKET, he could not cope.

A brother and sister, both endured the pressure of a life of trauma. One learned to empty their BUCKET and start to shine and regrettably, one did not.

THE DOWNWARD SPIRAL

As your BUCKET fills and your Diamond starts to lose its shine, what do you start to notice? There will come a point when you might start to feel yourself spiralling downwards and LIFE is not quite the same. There are different stages. At first you might feel like you have a load on your back, that something is weighing you down, and you feel heavy-hearted. I think we can all relate to that one. It can be a feeling that comes and goes at different times of life.

As you spiral down more, you start to feel infuriated. Not being able to function on all levels, energy is low, feeling tired a lot of the time, no longer firing on all cylinders.

Spiralling down further still, you start to feel a failure, the guilt for letting down family, friends, colleagues and your community to say nothing of yourself. At worst, that point when you hit rock bottom. We have worked with many clients that have shared with us, that they feel they are just existing. How many times have I heard 'I feel I don't want to get up in the morning'?

Well the good news is as I tell everyone, you have the power to put the brakes on and turn the spiral around. Not by someone else doing it for you or to you but by YOU doing it for YOURSELF – no talking, no medication, no effort! Imagine that – you can Heal Yourself!

> **'Remove stress from the body and**
> **the body regenerates itself.**
> **You can heal yourself.'**
>
> *Rhonda Byrne*
> *Author of 'The Secret'*

Caroline's Points to Ponder

1. On a scale of 1 to 10, how bright is your Diamond?

2. Do an analysis of the HISTORY that fills your BUCKET.

3. Where are you on that spiral downwards of LIFE?

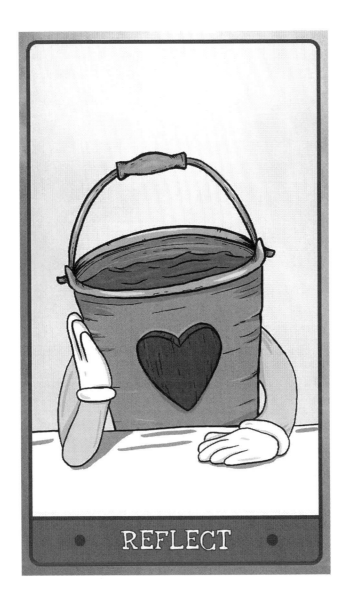

'*We either make
ourselves miserable
or make ourselves strong.
The amount of work is the same.*'

Carlos Castaneda
Best-selling author and anthropologist

Chapter Ten
The Roller Coaster Ride –
Go with the Flow
(Feel It to Heal It!)

Now you understand Diamonds and Buckets, the last thing we want to share with you is the ROLLER COASTER RIDE. Why? Because the journey to empty the BUCKET is a detox of the body.

Have you ever been on a roller coaster? Not everyone has. They are big scary things these days. On a day out my grandchildren would pull my hand and excitably say, 'Come on, Nanny, come on this with us!' What could I possibly say? 'OK then, let's go.' Whether with friends or family, I bet you share the same or similar experience. You queue up and pay your money, and next thing you are strapped in and only then does it hit you – there is no getting off until the ride has stopped!

So, someone delights in hitting the button then off you go. Scream, shout, screw up your eyes or have them wide open as you wave and hoot. There is nothing you can do whatever you feel until it stops and off you get. Your feet are back on the ground, maybe your legs are a bit wobbly, but there is a real buzz going on. Then you say to yourself, 'Wow, I did it, think I might even go on it again!'

Well there is no doubt about it that when you start to empty the BUCKET because of the HISTORY embedded in your body's muscle memory and begin to release, it is no easy ride. What has gone in has to come out. You have to 'Feel It to Heal It'; tensions, memories, feelings, emotions, and pain.

When you go on a roller coaster there are exciting moments and scary ones. You can feel exhilarated one minute and petrified the next. And so, it is when you go on the roller coaster of healing from your past.

A few years back I was so stunned when I was going through some old photographs and came across the picture I took years ago of my two youngest. We were on a roller coaster (only a little one by today's standards), and in one moment I turned around and took a photograph. Wow – did I ever think that image would say so much and serve me in my work years on! It illustrates our point completely. My daughter looks petrified and my son is exhilarated and excited. Magic! So, if you are going to heal your body, detox all your HISTORY to empty your BUCKET, then depending on what you have endured, you will wear one of two faces at different times. Not just one – but both. From your first Release session, the ride starts.

As I mentioned previously, if stuck in your BUCKET you will have five key Release experiences, whether that is in a practice session itself or in the days following as the body processes the information. Be very clear that whatever has gone into your BUCKET MUST come out at some point! The tension, memories, feelings, emotions, and pain.

Let me share examples of this from clients' experiences.

Tension

Everyone releases tension, that is the physical vibrating/tremoring of the body as it releases. Back pain is caused because of tension in the psoas. Many have sat up after the first session and said the pain has gone. One lady had been in a pain clinic for eight years with neck and shoulder pain. After her first session – gone! Many, many have that experience; blown away by the freedom of movement that comes from releasing tension from a level that no other can. The best prize of all is when breathing improves because tension has released from the psoas, which makes sense as it is attached to the diaphragm. With all that internal flinching, no wonder breath is taken away too.

We are all like coiled springs – so the body's vibrations enable the muscles to feel less tension and joints to feel freer. Bruxism (grinding of teeth) stops, for the tension around the jaw is released.

Memories

When memories surface, it is extraordinary. They can go back to the day of birth. Two stories that spring to mind relate to early childhood experiences.

Martin shared after his session that he felt scared as he saw a shadowed face but he could not see any detail. A hand was put to his throat, he was pinned to the wall and thought he was going to die. After he finished, I asked him if he recalled it as something from his childhood. He said quite emphatically it wasn't.

Martin was local and came to the weekly group session the following week. When it came to the sharing he said, 'Wow, I was about 11 and at school. I wanted to go into the classroom to get my bag. The teacher said no. When he was distracted, I snuck around to go and get my bag. He saw me, swung round, put his hand against my throat and pinned me to the wall. I saw his face, clear as anything. No wonder I have felt so angry all my life. No wonder I prefer to be outside in nature.'

I reminded him of the experience he had in the Workshop. It was incredible to see him put the pieces of the jigsaw together; that is what memories do. Memories that our body remembers but we do not, it seems almost unbelievable. For some people they are dreadful memories, but by being released, they clear the feelings and tension from the body. They make sense of life and why we are who we are as adults. Remember, our HISTORY forms us.

I am compelled to share two more stories. After her second session, Marcia was very emotional. She said she saw herself at two years old. Her grandfather was looking after her and her finger got cut off. She said it wasn't about the finger, as that was an accident. She said, 'What I saw were the images of all my family turning up and really have a go at my grandad. I always wondered why he kept his distance.' She had a realisation that for all her life she had no relationship with her grandad, and it was due to the fact that he was blamed for her accident. He was scared to be close to her for what had happened in the past. It gave her peace to know that it was not a personal thing. She understood and it allowed her to put closure on the whole situation.

Finally, there was Lynn, who had booked four sessions with her partner. On session three, she sat up and was sobbing. Her partner said, 'Are you OK?' I assured him that it was all part of her releasing. I asked if she wanted to talk about it. She said, 'Not with him here.' Her partner went into a side room. She shared the memories that came up for her was when she was three. She could see the older boys in the neighbourhood, sons of her parents' friends, and what they did to her. 'Now I realise I am like I am because of what happened. You are the first person to hear this.' I advised her to seek some counselling to help her process from this, but that it was good to come out. The following week, she was a different woman. She had shared with her partner and felt relief.

She called me some weeks later and said, 'You and TRE have changed my life. I am seeing a counsellor and I feel so different about myself.'

So many clients have their story of memories that go back to early years. Without TRE, they would never have been able to recall them and what is wonderful is they have understood not just more about themselves but also about their family, questioning what caused their father or their mother to reject them, to drink or be abusive or narcissistic? With those powerful insights comes a sense of forgiveness, acceptance and peace within.

Feelings

When guiding clients through to get used to the extraordinary power of the body, I say feelings can surface, either with memories or without. Feelings such as sadness, fear, hate, hurt, grief, guilt, anger, shame or anything else.

I have witnessed and supported many a client with the release of all their feeling. If the feelings are associated with childhood experiences, they may not always know that initially. The feeling is there but with no memory.

Let me share some examples. Chris was desperate for family unity. Having tried everything with her husband and two sons, nothing had made any impact. She was on the edge. I ran a private workshop for her, her husband, her sibling and their partner. There had been a big falling out with the other sibling.

During the second Release session, she whispered to me she felt angry. Her hands were clenched, but more than that, so were her teeth. The tension was so intense. I said to her, 'You need to release this anger, just let it out.' She certainly did! I was happy for her that she just let it go. It was no bad thing either that her family had a measure of just how much she had been holding. She felt a huge weight had been lifted. It was the start of an incredible healing journey for her.

I was working online with Francine, a young lady who lived in France. She was releasing and fear came up for her, then panic. My presence and guidance though online were reassuring enough that she finished the session. When the session was over, she shared that as a nine-year-old child she had an accident and was rushed to hospital. It was touch and go and she was lucky to be alive. She experienced all the feelings along with the memories she had at that time. Then it was gone!

I feel blessed to have been able to support those who have had their feelings emerge. Feelings from dark situations in their life including many that painfully go back to childhood.

Emotions

Feelings and memories, of course, can bring up the emotion too. Emotions can come up without memories, laughter, tears, sound. I will share something of them all.

Laughter impacts the lung meridian. The diaphragm is involved here and hence laughter frees up tension and breathing eases. The urge to laugh comes out of nowhere. In Workshops if one or two start to laugh, it is infectious. The craziest example was a chap called Pete whom I worked with online. For virtually the whole session he laughed, a constant hilarious kind of laugh. At one point I had to turn my mic off, for I was laughing too. I was reminded of when I was a child putting my penny in the slot machine in the amusements on the seafront – the Laughing Policeman – always had us in stitches! Pete said after that he felt amazing but I was not surprised!

As my mother used to say, 'All that laughter, it will only lead to tears,' and that stands true in releasing. Tears can be felt as a trickle or a complete outpouring. There are so many (mostly men) who have shed no tears since childhood, so it is wonderful when suppressed emotions come through. This has happened so often for men. An actor attended my course. (I have had various performers and artists.) He happened to be from one of my favourite drama series. I never told him that, because he was there not as an actor but as himself. I sat and held his hand whilst he released the tears from his childhood.

When tears came for Brian, it was for the first time he could ever remember, and he shared that he had been saying to himself for all his years, 'Why did he [his father] do that to me, the man, now I am saying, why did he do that to me, the child?' He told me that for all the beatings he got as a lad, he was never going to show his emotion. He had held onto it for all those years.

Grief, when it releases, is incredibly moving. The outpouring of emotion as the tears flow, because the body is letting go, brings such relief. Releasing grief is so important for anyone but especially for the elderly, as it sets them free of their mental and emotional pain. They often hold on to so much, especially if having cared for their partner, sometimes for years. It puts a strain on their own health. To see them smile again and find peace from their grief is a reward like no other.

Nancy was a lovely elderly lady who was quite scared in her first session. She didn't like the feeling of her body shaking but managed to get through. She was grief-stricken over the recent loss of her husband of many years. Having cared for him for a long time, her emotions were suppressed. She cried.

But the lovely thing is she called me next morning and said she was out in her garden, the sun was shining, she looked up to the sky with her hands together as in prayer, raised them up and said to herself, 'Now what shall I do first?' All of a sudden, she started to shake. I asked her what she did, and she replied, 'I just let it happen!' I was so proud of her. She then made me laugh as she said she was tempted to go and pour a gin and tonic!

Pain

The body does indeed remember pain; from old injuries, accidents, operations, or anything else one might have experienced. Clients have experienced pain sensations in the wrist, elbow, knee, ankle, hip, back, shoulder, neck. Birth pains too either from giving birth or one's own birth.

In her first session, Sue was crying, gagging and feeling scared. I held her hand to support her (always with permission), as she was clearly going through something very challenging. This lasted for quite a few minutes. She also broke wind. She finally stretched out. When she sat up and felt ready, she told me that not so long ago she was taken by ambulance to hospital and they tried to put a tube down her throat, and she went through the whole scenario in that physical release. She even broke wind in the ambulance, and she said they all laughed. Incredible! What goes in has to come out.

Now you can start to see how much of a roller coaster this can be? I tell everyone they have to 'Feel It to Heal It' – when it is gone, it is gone. Not temporarily but forever, totally life-changing, transformational.

Sound

The final thing that can come up in a Release session is sound. We can lose our voice in childhood. From throwaway comments like 'children should be seen and not heard', 'you're only a child' or 'you have nothing worth saying' to the worst kind of childhood traumas where a child grows up petrified to say anything for fear of reprisal. The voice gets suppressed.

The most extraordinary sound was Chris who attended a Derby Workshop. She started to make a wolf-like sound. It was extraordinary, very primordial and it went on for a while. She had no idea where it had come from and yet after it was over she felt quite remarkable.

From gurgling to yelling to shouting out, the voice finds its way back. Sound, of course, is a vibration so clients who have a tight throat are encouraged to make sound which is often enough to make a shift. Very profound.

Other experiences on the roller coaster can be tiredness, weird dreams and possible disturbed sleep. If one has had anxiety, panic attacks or even suicidal thoughts, they will at some point be re-experienced. But we educate everyone to know how to deal with what comes up.

To sum up the Roller Coaster, the benefits, challenges and resilience are all there, dipping in and out. The great thing is you don't have to wait to empty the bucket of the negatives before we experience the benefits. The resilience kicks in quickly. When women email in and share that they find themselves saying 'No' or dealing with situations very differently, and not being fazed in the usual way, I feel so pleased for them – it is just great.

Layer by layer, the body heals, and every time the body releases, the Diamond gets a bit more shine. The more the shine, the more transformation is experienced.

'Once you start approaching your body with curiosity rather than fear, everything shifts.'

Bessel van der Kolk
Psychiatrist and best-selling author of 'The Body Keeps the Score'

Caroline's Points to Ponder

1. Have you ever had a healing crisis experience?

2. Are you emotional and do you know why?

3. Do you have a feeling of something suppressed in your body?

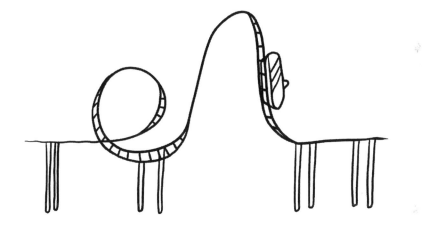

'Somewhere, something incredible is waiting to be known.'

Carl Sagan
*Astronomer, scientist, author and presenter
of most-watched American TV series, Cosmos*

Part III – Taking Responsibility to Discover the Power Within
Chapter Eleven
Proof of the Pudding – Gary's Story

T he scene has been set. I have shared with you the underlying principles of our message. What really drives my passion is the magic that happens from doing the practice.

Gary's story is a great example of the many aspects of healing that can happen. I was at a friend's party one night, mingling and striking up a conversation with a stranger. A common question that I always get asked is '…and what do you do?' So, I told them! Then someone tapped me on the shoulder and asked if we could chat. He had heard what I did and wanted to know more.

Gary was 53 years old, married with two children and worked as a policeman/social worker. He told me he was feeling the impact of stress and anxiety. One of Gary's traumas was an assault where he was nearly kicked to death by a soldier and his friends, when he had gone to help them.

He had tried all sorts of therapies and treatments to overcome or deal with his high stress levels. I asked him if he would like to join my group that was starting the following week to which he responded with enthusiasm that he would. Timing is everything.

When he first arrived at the studio, he was putting his shoes in the rack and said to me, 'If you can sort my stress out, you will be the first!' No pressure then! With my faith in the practice, I was not fazed. There were four in the group. As I gave my pre-talk, Gary looked petrified. His eyes were like a rabbit in headlights, so much so that I thought he was going to run from the room. I kept a very close eye on him throughout the session. He managed to get through the Release session. Afterwards he shared that he felt very calm.

He told me during the week that he really enjoyed the session after a wobbly start. He wondered if I had noticed that he was nearly sick as I was giving my talk at the beginning regarding letting the stresses out. This had been a feature in his life, especially if doing any public speaking. He felt he had been covering up his stress for so long that it would only take a small thing to give him a panic attack.

> In the email, he wrote: *I am glad I didn't run for the exit, as that evening I felt somehow calmer about my worries and could put them to one side to enjoy an evening with my family and did not feel the need to hide from the worries with a glass or two of wine, as usual. I did have a glass later on and instead of it making me feel tired and detached, I felt quite chatty and cheeky (like I used to be!) and my other half wondered what had happened to me! I also slept better that night and my back pain was less than usual in the morning. I found myself having some quite vivid dreams.*
>
> *Although a bit upset after the session, I think it was tears of happiness, as previously I really thought I was dying, having been in such pain all day and night for five years – nobody can understand how that feels unless you have had it! I have been referred by my GP to a rheumatology specialist as she suspected I could be developing early onset Parkinson's, but I do not even think it is worth keeping the appointment now, I will have a think about that.*

Such positive reactions from one 20-minute release!

He attended regularly for six sessions. Every week he would email me and let me know what was changing for him. Week on week, there was always a noticeable shift as layer by layer he was healing.

His mental health was improving, and his energy levels were increasing. He was thinking much more positively (as he always used to). Despite the daily stresses, he felt he was back to his old self and able to deal with it and more importantly, able to separate it from his home life.

He told me: *'My muscles are less stiff, and the pain is reduced. My stomach is less bloated and the pressure and pain in my solar plexus had reduced by far. My appetite had started to return, and I am not feeling sick or anxious anymore. During the week I was able to do so many things I had not been able to do since being ill, and my memory was beginning to function again.*

I had patience with the kids and my boss had noticed my creativity returning at work. My eyes are not hurting anymore. Before just looking at people, I had to drop my gaze after a short time, as the muscles behind my eyes would hurt so much. I could not cope with light very well and struggled to see in normal light as it hurt my eyes. This is improving and my night vision is coming back too. I can turn my head without pain now and my injured back is not hurting as much at all. I am also sleeping better, and some nights manage to sleep for seven hours without waking, unheard of for many years.

My skin is less oily, my nasal passages are clearing, I have my sense of smell back. I have got my mojo back and at work my boss noticed the difference, saying I seem to be more focused and committed than normal!

All my symptoms are nearly a thing of the past and I am feeling so happy to be feeling better, and yet sad that I had wasted so many years of my life being ill. I found myself sad for my family and friends as well as the family I was not able to support as I would have liked to.

So for me, this has given me my life back, my family their dad back and my friends their cheeky happy-go-lucky mate back!

It was this sharing of Gary's most detailed healing that more than blew me away. I felt so privileged to be the initiator of his healing journey. It made me realise many things but mostly that the human body is truly incredible. If this was my earliest experience, witnessing such profound change, what else was I going to discover?

Eight years later

Gary has dipped in and out of group sessions over the years. We have chatted on the phone now and again and of course he has had more ups and downs in life to deal with. When I started to write this chapter, I thought to myself, 'I wonder how Gary is doing now?' so I jumped up out of my chair and called him. He was pleased I called and told me he had been thinking of me too and was going to call. He was still doing his practice – can you image my joy! Nearly eight years on, he still had a clear message – keep going. He wanted to meet up and said, 'I honestly believe this prevented my onset Parkinson's and it is this I want to share. The Parkinson's organisation should know about this.'

Unfortunately, COVID-19 had us all in lockdown by the end of that week, so the meeting never happened. Something we look forward to when we are free.

> **'The proof of the pudding is in the eating. By a small sample we may judge of the whole piece.'**
>
> *Miguel de Cervantes*
> *Author of 'Don Quixote'*

Caroline's Points to Ponder

1. Do you feel the impact of stress and anxiety from your work?

2. Do you drink to hide worries?

3. How many of Gary's symptoms are you impacted by too?

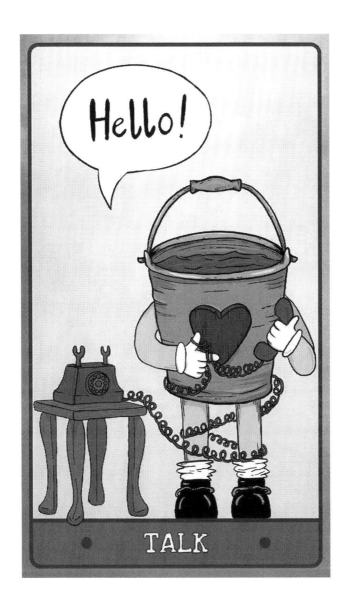

'Help, don't hurt.
Teach, don't tell.
Show, don't shame.
Parent, don't punish.
Our world needs more
heart-whole adults,
not more refugees from
childhood.'

L. R Knost
Author and Social Justice Activist,
Director of children's rights group

Chapter Twelve
The Impact of Childhood Trauma –
When ACEs are High

The all-important American study of 17,000 adults on the impact of Adverse Childhood Experiences (ACE)* concluded that the higher the ACEs, the more likely there would be health issues in adult life that would lead to premature death. Experiences such as neglect, abandonment or abuse, growing up around drugs, alcohol, having one or no parents, or one who has been incarcerated or had committed suicide. There is so much more. I very soon realised how true this was. The majority of those I have taught to Release presented with physical, mental and/or emotional pain from their childhood experiences.

The more my clients have shared, the more I have understood just how much of a silent killer stress is. It eats away at you. For those who have discovered what their body can do, miracles happen in different ways. Indeed, as van de Kolk says, 'the Body Keeps the Score'. But it doesn't need to, as Michael and Leila testify.

The impact of boarding school

I spent 12 years teaching in a secondary-level boarding school. The pupils' parents were in the military so many lived abroad. I joined the staff the year after they went co-ed. It took some years for the girls to be accepted and respected. That aside, it was clear that some students loved the life.

* *The CDC-Kaiser Permanente Adverse Childhood Experiences (ACE) Study is one of the largest investigations of childhood abuse and neglect and household challenges and later-life health and well-being. The original ACE Study was conducted at Kaiser Permanente from 1995 to 1997 with two waves of data collection.*

There were others, however, that didn't. For many, it was tough at the age of 11, leaving home, parents, family, friends and in many respects, their freedom. No wonder there were so many tears as they struggled to settle in. The house parents had a challenging role. I saw children and teenagers go through some harrowing experiences during that time. Still today I wonder just how much of an impact it had on their well-being in adult life. I was informed of the suicide of an ex-pupil who was only in her twenties. When I read the story, all the signs were there – boarding school, divorced parents, debt, low self-esteem and the torment of social media. Her BUCKET was full and she had no Release.

What has been your experience of boarding school?

Take a moment to jot down your thoughts.

Michael's Story

Michael was in his early thirties, a young family man with a career. He had suffered anxiety until about the age of 17. He then got on with his life, went to university, was successful in his work, married and had two children. Life was good. But then he started to suffer severe anxiety. He attended a Workshop to learn to Release. He was quite stunned by the power of his body. But like all with childhood experiences, it was only the start of his healing journey; the impact of early years would show up. From his many communications, he shared this:

> I cried a lot when I first went to boarding school as I didn't want to be there. You feel like you are abandoned by the people you love most and the emotional safety net of home is ripped from below you and you lose all that stability. But then you give up crying as you realise that no one is going to come and help you or take you back home, not even your parents as they sent you there!

> So, you lock away these feelings as showing them is weakness and you need to learn to survive alone, no matter what it takes. Sounds crazy saying this about a school that people are paying hundreds of thousands of pounds to send children to. But in some cases, it is like living (being locked up) with the

people that bully you every day! So you essentially 'freeze' and that is what happened to me from the age of nine/ten.

He was glad to get that off his chest. Michael's sharing is a profound insight into the experience that thousands of children have had in their life. When I talk to staff at boarding schools, I always share Michael's experience.

He contacted me again some weeks later.

I have had OCD in relationships, questioning relationships, questioning sexuality and constantly checking everything was locked. These issues are much better now as I now really see them as OCD rather than me genuinely questioning these aspects of my life. This has meant that they have greatly reduced. I am more positive and much more emotionally aware.

I never cried this much and it is what I wanted when I started the process.

The interesting thing is that I had a profound crying session and I experienced some things that were different. Normally I would just cry, with no thoughts or memories, maybe just little ones. This time when I was crying, I felt like I was lying in my dorm bed at boarding school and really started to cry for my mother. I began to question what the hell my mum did and how she could have done that to me. Why did she abandon me?

There was nothing about my dad as I never really saw him anyway as he worked a lot, but when we did see him he was always in a very bad mood and not nice at all really. Mum was the one that I was close to and I felt these feelings of disappointment and sadness that she would do this to me. It felt very real, and then when the feeling had gone, and I stood up, I felt like I became that nine-year-old that was sent away to school and saw the world as him for a couple of minutes; then this went and I felt much, much better! It was almost like the nine-year-old in me had at last been able to come out after being locked away for so long. He was allowed to feel the sadness of that moment, and the element of me that had been cut off had been able to re-join, making me more whole.

Following this, I had a strong desire to increase my spiritual practice and began to mediate for 20 to 30 minutes a day. My practice had greatly reduced over time to maybe 10 minutes a day, and now I have really begun to be more present. I thought I was mindful and a conscious (in the spiritual way) person, but it has become very apparent that I am not at all! This has been really amazing and by practising this daily, I am beginning to see life very differently.

Michael's story gives a real insight to the feelings and emotions that get locked in the body of a child. He has set that little boy free and no longer carries the pain.

Maybe his story resonates with you or you know someone who has yet to set their inner child free?

Leia's Story – a mother's neglect

Leia attended a workshop presenting with PTSD. She shares her story:

The stresses of being a student, mother and being unemployed for a number of months had made my life very challenging in recent years, before and after my PTSD diagnosis. With complex childhood trauma, I found even the smallest tasks very difficult in my life and was consumed by anxiety in attempting them.

I had tried psychotherapy, EMDR* and hypnotherapy, and although helpful in relieving some of these issues, this was never long-term and relied on me attending expensive appointments which were not as cathartic to me as the Total Release Experience® which was something I was interested to discover. What I love about the practice is that you are taught to allow 'an all-over body experience' to change the physiology of your mind. It gives your body the opportunity to take its power back and help you trust in the body's wisdom to heal you.

Doing the practice has given me insights into the source of some of my major issues, some going as far back as when I was a baby.

* *See glossary at the back for the full meaning.*

I have been able to access memories which have been particularly enlightening for me, though not very pleasant! I feel recently that I have been shaking from 'the cot' which has been quite extraordinary. My mother neglected me as a baby so much that my tremors at the moment feel like they are resonating from this, but it's taken me a number of weeks to access them.

Usually we approach these issues with our minds first and the body later, if at all. When our minds approach our issues, we can override our emotions, rationalising our feelings. But when our body accesses emotions first, we do not have the opportunity to explain them away. Instead in the TRE the body takes over releasing trapped emotions by over-riding any interference from our minds. The result is a deep psychotherapeutic work on the purest level of the body wisdom we all share. It has helped me feel much more confident as a powerful collaborator in my own continual recovery, and this has had a profound effect on my belief to heal myself, which is exactly what the TRE has allowed me to start doing, only this time for keeps. Now any time I feel anxious, I Release. Afterwards my feelings of anxiety disappear, and I feel more capable. I also have managed to avoid some PTSD symptoms that usually mean I get ill when my uni assignments are due. That did not happen this year which was such a relief so I will keep practising it!

I would recommend the Total Release Experience® to EVERYBODY: man, woman and child. It is a thoroughly effective technique which is empowering and healing. It is not always easy to do and can be challenging when it brings up memories we have forgotten. It may seem illogical to those who want to pin down how it works, but the rewards in trusting your body through the process are so immense, that it is simply a gift that none of us should live without.

A gift indeed. Michael and Leia are just two of so many cases where the body has healed itself. No matter what you hold on to, you can set yourself free.

'Healing is the end of conflict with yourself.'

Stephanie Gailing
Astrologer, well-being coach and author

Caroline's Points to Ponder

1. How high are the ACEs you recall from your own childhood?

2. Did you go to boarding school? Was it a happy time or something else?

3. Did you ever feel neglected as a child? How did you cope?

4. What impact has childhood experiences had on your adult health and life?

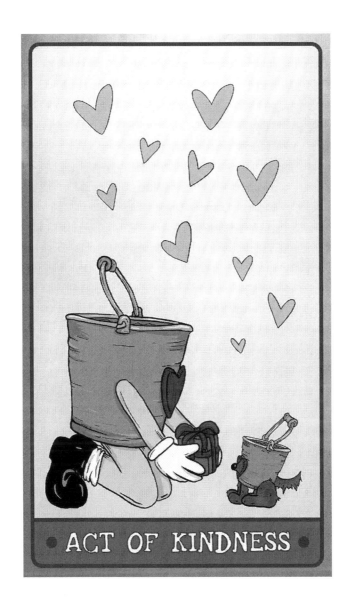

'Anything that is "wrong"
with you began
as a survival mechanism
in childhood.'

Dr Gabor Maté
Canadian psychologist and best-selling author of
'When the Body Says No'

Chapter Thirteen
Hearing Lost in Childhood – Angharad's story

There is nothing more wonderful than when someone discovers for themselves, through their releasing, just how their early years trauma shaped them and impacted them for the whole of their life. Even more profound is knowing that as their body releases and the trauma reveals itself, it puts pieces of the jigsaw together.

Angharad had a difficult childhood; she suffered abuse and was a frightened child. She used to have nightmares and felt terrified most of the time. She had suffered from hearing loss since an early age and for a while had a hearing aid. The trauma of her childhood had made her simply shut down her hearing, as she could not take any more of the shouting and anger in the family home.

By the time she was a teenager, she had become depressed, disconnected, and disassociated, and suffered from PTSD. For many of her teenage years and during her twenties, she was in a state of hyper-vigilance and stress. Her inner tension would recreate scenarios confirming to her that the world was unsafe, she could not trust anyone, and she ended up taking substances that would help her to escape from her trauma. She developed a mask, so others had no idea about the difficulties she was feeling inside. Angharad spent most of her youth out of her body and was completely ungrounded, so she did not have to feel what her body was telling her. She was too frightened to heal as she was in denial about the things that had happened to her.

In her twenties she was re-traumatising herself by having powerful healings yet was still unable to come back fully into her body to feel grounded. She was afraid of the huge fear and anxiety that was buried deep inside, like a volcano about to erupt… and erupt it did!

Just before she turned 40, she had a major life change and left the father of her children. It felt like the rug had been pulled from under her, as he had been her safety net. She developed a nervous twitch, began having panic attacks, and was constantly anxious. She eventually met her new husband and started to feel safe around male energy for the first time in her life. But it was a year or two later she began to have what she thought were crazy experiences, thinking that she was going mad. Her body was reacting, feeling cold with pins and needles, and uncontrollable shaking and tremoring – this would last for about half an hour three or four times a day.

Someone guided her to one of my Workshops and then she started to make sense of her experiences. At one point she had a big release of crying and sobbing as if her heart would break. When she was a little girl, she had never cried and as a young adult she would have outbursts of rage and anger instead of crying. It was as if she had forgotten how to cry and was scared of crying.

However, Angharad made that classic mistake of feeling good so stopped her practice, but in a few months started struggling to hear again, feeling like she was under water, so she decided to return to her releasing practise. Before she started the next session, she set an intention to let go of whatever was causing the hearing loss.

After two sessions her stress levels went up, and she struggled to communicate with her husband. She felt distress every time he tried to communicate with her. The overwhelming feeling she had, that she could not take anymore, was how she felt as a child and she knew she was projecting her feelings towards her father onto her husband.

Despite the releasing being felt in her head, there was still no change with her hearing, so she went to get her ears checked and washed out at the doctors.

Angharad continues with her incredible story: *The nurse found an object in my right ear and pulled it out! It was a small piece of white plastic with a silver wire sticking out! I was shocked! How on earth did that get in there?! I had had my ears checked for years and nothing had been found before.*

I mentioned this to my father later on in the day and he was shocked. He told me that when I was eight years old I had a grommet inserted in my ear, but the operation had failed. The doctors had searched for the grommet but could not find it, and told my parents that it had fallen out. I then went on to have a hearing aid. I went online and googled grommets and yes indeed the object that the nurse had pulled out was the grommet, 34 years later! I can now hear out of my right ear!

I know that as well as releasing the stress and trauma from the operation, and the trauma of not wanting to hear my father shouting, the releasing had also brought the grommet to the surface to be released, by the rhythmic rocking motion of the head. I feel my eight-year-old girl body had not wanted the operation to work as she was terrified at the thought of hearing and caused my body to hide the grommet. The Total Release Experience® has changed my life. It has changed the way I see and relate to the world.

I was quite astounded by this wonderful story as others have been as I shared it. It is testimony as to the importance of our message, that the regularity is key. If Angharad had not re-engaged with the practice, she would never have regained her hearing.

'Experience has taught us that we have only one enduring weapon in our struggle against mental illness: the emotional discovery and emotional acceptance of the truth in the individual and unique history of our childhood.'

Alice Miller
Psychologist, psychoanalyst and author of
'The Drama of the Gifted Child'

Caroline's Points to Ponder

1. Do you recall 'shouting' adults when you were a child?

2. What did you do? How did you deal with it?

3. Do you feel childhood experiences have impacted your health in any way?

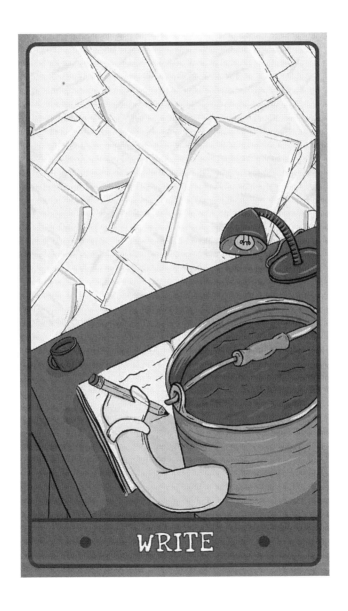

*'You must find the place
inside yourself
where nothing is impossible.'*

Deepak Chopra
Best-selling author and alternative medicine advocate

Chapter Fourteen
What Goes In Has to Come Out –
More Insights into the
Power of Healing

Phobias

I remember as a child being afraid of the dark. How many of us have a fear of something, whether that is spiders, water, confined spaces, crowds or any number of things? Take a moment to jot down the things you fear.

The practice has helped so many get over their fears. Here I share Vincent's healing experience from fear of flying.

We have just returned from holiday and had a very good time. I wanted to share that normally I am a very nervous experience flying, even with very mild turbulence. Last year, I attended a BA course 'Flying with Confidence' which helped but not that much.

On this occasion, however, the days before flying both out and on return I had practiced my releasing, and I was so very surprised as the result was outstanding. On both trips, I felt very relaxed and calm and when at one point we experienced strong turbulence for a few seconds, I practiced the relaxation exercises you showed me, as the result was very good. So thank you very much!

Health Anxiety

Dom was in a bad way when I met him. I visited him at his home to chat about what I could do to help him release from his anxiety.

He rarely visited the doctor, but out of nowhere and due to personal reasons, he was struck down with severe anxiety attacks. He began suffering with health anxiety which led to him being confined to home and off work. His weight fell from 11 stone 3lbs to 9 stone 12lbs, and he was unable to sleep, as his anxiety attacks increased. His health deteriorated.

He was convinced he was going to die from a heart attack, as his mother had. No end of times he was taken by ambulance to hospital. He agreed to come to the studio and committed to learn the programme.

He completed four sessions before he was forced to stop due to unrelated stomach problems. During this period, I continued to contact him with encouragement and told him not to let his mind control his body. With this in mind, he agreed to return to the group and finish his six sessions. More importantly, he started to practice twice a week at home.

> Dom says: *There were many times when I didn't feel like it but I knew it was starting to relax me and my mind.*
>
> *Three months on, I have been back at work for five weeks, my sleep has improved, and I no longer have anxiety attacks. My weight is now only 4lbs off my starting weight and whilst I have not fully recovered, the turnaround has been dramatic, and my friends and family cannot believe my progress. My advice to anybody else suffering in a similar manner is not to give up hope.*

Pinpointing issues

Seeing the results he was getting, Dom's wife Pat attended sessions too. A month or two after her course, an email arrived out of the blue:

> *Pat has asked me to share this with you. It could be that the TRE not only heals the body but also pinpoints the problem area.*

She has just spoken to the doctor and it's her left ovary that has the 'complex cyst' on it.

This means that when she was doing her releasing and her body kept gravitating towards the left and up into her pelvic/ovary area, it somehow knew there was something wrong!! She asked me to tell you that she feels this is a real breakthrough!

Letting go of a traumatic past

Kelly was encouraged to get in touch by her doctor. She called me and asked if she could attend an upcoming Workshop but her concern was that she was wheelchair-bound. I asked her what happened. She told me that her sister was murdered and she herself had jumped from the top floor of a burning house. Trauma had impacted her life for 20 years. It was the trauma in her body that needed to release.

We managed to get Kelly into a place that she could hopefully release, supported by cushions. She did and her healing journey began.

She shared with me what has changed for her:

After just a couple of Release sessions at home, there was a huge shift in my brain. I have spent my entire adult life living in the past, being hurt, angry, wanting revenge and justice for my sister. The pain and guilt just would not go!

I now know that I was actually holding on to the hurt, pain, anger and guilt because I was too afraid of what would happen if I did let it go. I have spent 20 years in and out of therapy. I have had every talking therapy there is, including EMDR, but they all have left me even more angry and confused.

Doing the TRE at home, completely on my own, with no talking, no interruptions, no force and no "appointment time", has been astounding. I cried so much I thought I could never stop. I allowed it to all come out, whenever and however it wanted to.

The result? I am leaving the past where it belongs. I cannot change what has happened, nor can I change what will happen in the future. The only person I was hurting was myself. The anger has gone, the guilt has gone. I don't feel quite so afraid of the world anymore. I'm doing OK. I'm crying writing this as I can't believe how far I have come in a few short months, when no one has been able to help me in decades.

I still struggle with PTSD, but I like to think I'm beating it, instead of it beating me! Grateful thanks.

Healing from pain

I had never thought about the word 'pain' until I read a book called *The Story of Pain* by Joanna Bourke. Gosh, what does it mean exactly! In her book, Joanna quotes Dr Peter Mere Latham, who was Queen Victoria's personal physician:

Things which all men know infallibly by their own perceptive experience, cannot be made plainer by words. Therefore, let Pain be spoken of simply as Pain.

Our body remembers pain and it is extraordinary how pain has been felt and then released either in a session or in the processing afterwards, from old accidents, injuries, operations and even birth pains.

Those in pain clinic suffer because there is no cure. The tension in the body is causing their pain. I recall a lady who had been in pain clinic for over seven years. At the end of her first session, she declared her neck pain had released. It never returned.

Pain in legs and knees

Gill shares: I have tried all sorts of 'healing' methods and most worked, in some way. But nothing has helped me as reliably, and cost effectively, as the Total Release Experience®.

It started with immediate effect after the Workshop of being pain free in my legs and knees (I have been in pain for two years following an injury) and continued with the wonderful feeling of release and calmness after a 'session' at home. This is an amazing tool to heal, shield and prepare.

And hip!

In Manchester, there was a good-sized group. Tim sat up after the first session which had been quite emotional for him. He said: *I do not wish to sound evangelical, but eight months ago a car drove through my house. I have had hip pain ever since. Despite all sorts of treatments and MRI scans, nothing has touched it. But now it has gone!* It was quite moving to hear him share this experience.

Michelle's unexpected miracle healing

I attended a Workshop with no real expectation. We went along to simply explore something that sounded interesting, but we were not prepared for it to impact on us in the way that it did.

I was sceptical, because for me I believed that therapeutic change (especially linked to trauma) is the result of interventions such as talking therapies, EMDR and medication.

After the Workshop, which was incredibly powerful, I felt tired yet relaxed and felt this was something I could take into my practice as a way of releasing the build-up of stress. I felt so relaxed – it was a strange feeling, almost light and floaty. About a week after the first practice I noticed I wasn't in so much pain. The things I was experiencing were not what I expected at all.

In 2004 I suffered an injury to my cervical and lumbar spine. I had spells in a wheelchair, six surgeries, five of which were major and could have resulted in paralysis. I lost my job within a mental health ward and suffered low mental health: the impact on my family was huge. Over time and with each surgery, my mobility enabled me to get my life back to a stage of being able to re-train as a psychotherapist, enter the workforce, drive and enjoy life. However, I still was reliant on medication on a daily basis and I suffered a lot of migraines.

I also had a history of trauma. I had been in a traumatic relationship and suffered seven childhood Adverse Childhood Experiences, so my body was holding past and present trauma which I didn't realise, despite over 140 hours of psychotherapy as part of my clinical training and Master's degree course. On an intellectual level, I felt my past had been dealt with successfully.

In the weeks after the Workshop, I realised that I wasn't in so much pain. The improvement was gradual over the course of about six weeks. It started that I missed my lunch meds, followed by teatime meds, then I didn't need amitriptyline every night to sleep, finally lowering my overall dose to about 25% of my original medication doses. I also now have spells of being completely pain-free – something I haven't felt for over 15 years! I can only put this down to the practice of the TRE, nothing else changed. I had no other therapy at this time. I now only get a prescription every 10/12 weeks instead of every 4 weeks on the dot. This practice has changed my life!

Low back pain is so common. Despite the money spent on looking for relief, when clients learn to Release, the first thing that seems to go is back pain. Back pain is tension in the psoas, so there is no way to access it. Sciatica too is healed very quickly.

Returning back to what he loved

When I met Lewis at a Workshop, I was taken aback by his story. He was a young man who had worked for many years as a community mental health nurse. He was feeling the impact of stress and was beginning to spiral downwards. The only way out he could see for himself was to give up the work he loved. It had taken its toll on his physical, mental, and emotional well-being. He was suffering from social anxiety and desperate for something that might work for him. It was after lunch on that day he said to me 'Amazing, I have social anxiety and yet I have just been outside and have been talking to people.' He left that day full of hope.

I was so thrilled to hear from Lewis a couple of months later:

I just want to let you know that I have felt so much better since the Workshop. I have been on the roller coaster, feeling so drained and tired. I had to go into A & E on Monday because my heart was pounding and getting pains. I do have a recent heart condition, thickening of heart, so that may have contributed to it. All the tests were fine. I am feeling less tired now. I also had some aches and pains spontaneously in lower back and hamstring. They have all gone.

I am really very positive about life and optimistic about the future. I have done a couple of bar shifts and I am enquiring about agency work as a nurse. It is amazing!

I want my wife to do this, but she is reluctant. She has anxiety and does not love herself or believe in herself which she should as she is beautiful, clever, and funny.

Thanks for this and for teaching people to get back to homeostasis, to being able to enjoy life and shine like a diamond.

Lewis is now back as a Community Mental Health Nurse and his wife did attend to learn herself! How wonderful they have turned their own lives around by taking back control of their own well-being!

I give the last word here to Maria, one of many who have learnt to reconnect with their own body.

I did a short spontaneous session and it revealed something very new for me.

I am now waking up early in the morning feeling refreshed after a good night's sleep and I can get through the day without needing a nap. My body seems so much lighter as if a heavy load had been lifted (it has!). This is a particularly feel-good factor. I know sunny warm days help usually but I truly hope this will be lasting for me.

I feel hungry most of the time and since I am at home on my own, I am now cooking for myself. It is not new to me to have an ongoing conversation with my body, but now I am relieved we are listening to each other even more.

The bucket is finally emptying, thank heavens. I want to continue to have a friendship with my whole self-esteem, body, mind, heart and spirit.

Our body is the only place that we have to live – it makes sense to look after it! No matter what is going on in your body, when you learn to trust yourself and reconnect with what nature gave you – miracles can be yours too.

'If you are searching for that one person who will change your life, take a look in the mirror.'

Roman Price
Blogger and LifePulp Founder

Caroline's Points to Ponder

1. If you have anxiety, can you identify the main trigger?

2. What do you hold onto from the past that leaves you struggling to move forward?

3. Where do you feel the pain in your body? Do you really know what caused it, or did it creep up on you?

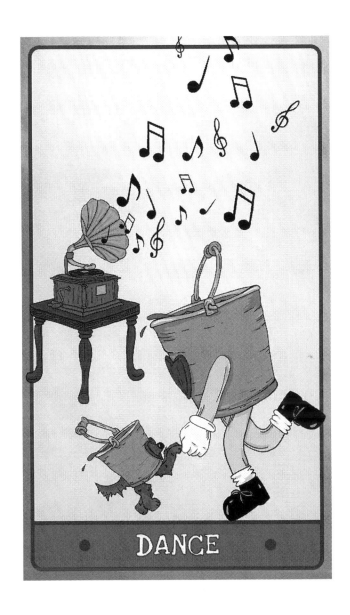

*'I cannot do all the good
that the world needs.
But the world needs all
the good I can do.'*

Jana Stanfield
Musician and motivational speaker

Chapter Fifteen
We are all Human –
Heroes and...

I had no doubt from the start of my journey that this would be the perfect practice for the service sector, be that the Fire, Military, Police, Ambulance and Prison Services, for two reasons. First, it is an empowering, cost-effective stress release programme and secondly, it requires no talking. In my early years, I had various clients from the service sectors come to my sessions. But breaking through to management has been a bigger challenge than I first thought. I shall start with the first of our Heroes.

The Fire Service

The Fire Service have the most stressful job in civilian society. They never know what they will encounter every time they go on a 'shout'. In 2015, I worked with my first firefighter. Amongst other things, he was dealing with back pain. After a few weeks of yoga classes, I asked him about his stress levels given his work. He was not giving much away, but he did say he had issues, admitting it was not the sort of conversation anyone had at work. He then signed up for a course of the TRE. He released emotions, memories and all that was his to Release. His back healed and he was in a better place when he finished. As much as I would have loved him to share with his colleagues – it was never going to happen. However, I wasn't going to give up that easily!

In 2016 another client worked in a marketing role for the Fire Service. She created an opportunity for me to deliver a presentation at the headquarters. I was excited and thought this was going to be the breakthrough I was looking for, as I stood in front of at least 25 personnel. Whilst my message was being delivered, you could hear a pin drop. Afterwards some came over and thought it would be great for someone they knew who would love to do it but only if the Service paid for it. I realised pretty quickly that most were in denial, either not recognising the impact of stress on themselves, or wanting someone else to invest in their well-being. Ironically, I heard some six months on that the firefighter who organised the talk was now off with stress!

In 2018 one of my practitioners in training had a firefighter friend who attended her case study group. I had a phone call one Sunday morning from a lady who herself was a firefighter and was excited that the man in question was 'transformed'. As a Well-being Champion, she wanted to know more. I offered her a free place on a course so she could experience it enough to be able to report back. She started the course and got amazing results but by session four she had a back injury and was off work, but I was not giving up! We kept in touch and she spoke to many people about it.

Eventually Daniel and I were invited to meet and present a strategy in 2018 to Senior Management dealing with well-being. This was unexpected and exciting. We went along to the headquarters and had a very productive meeting. What they loved about our work was the fact that it was both cost-effective compared to other services they were using as well as empowering personnel to start taking responsibility. The impression was that mental health in the Service was fast becoming a costly problem and nothing was changing.

A pilot Workshop was organised in October 2018 with Champions within the Service as well as admin staff and psychologists. We received very positive feedback and following on from this, the word started to spread. There were some who connected with it and healed, and some who thought they didn't need it. Then there were some who could not be bothered. Each to his own!

We have learned a lot from working with the Fire Service. One client reinforced what we were sharing in our message. A mutual friend had told him about our work two years previously. When he attended a Workshop with colleagues, I asked why it had taken so long to connect to it. He said, 'Well I am a fireman!' 'So, why now?' I asked, 'What is going on for you?' He replied, 'I am having difficult problems in my personal relationships; my eye is twitching, and I am stuttering.' There was more. This man would jump in the sea every day for the cold treatment and spend endless hours at the gym. That is not living, that is surviving!

He shared too, that in a day's work, all firefighters deal with trauma. When their shift is over, they go home and open the front door and say, 'Hello kiddies, Daddy's home!' but most are just wearing a painted smile. That said it all really. If the truth was known, there are a lot of painted smiles out there. Next time you see a firefighter – look in the eyes.

Of all the shared testimonials, this says it all!

I joined the Kent Fire and Rescue Service in 1994 aged 23. At the time I felt invincible, as you do, being a young man. Life and my career ticked by, experiencing good and bad incidents. I never really noticed any mental challenges. It was in 2003 that my life seemed to be going great and then suddenly, 'Crash!' What should normally be the highlight of one's career – pulling someone alive from a burning building – actually left me broken due to the conditions we endured. I had counselling not knowing what to expect and I felt worse from it, as I never found answers, but believed it was making me better, as I felt I could now cope. What I know now is time and my natural body made it easier, rather than the process or help I received.

As years moved on, all was fine until January 2019. A series of events left me in a very bad way, feeling immense anger, breaking down in tears for what would be the simplest of issues, thinking of suicide. Yes, I would say I was at rock bottom and at that crossroads – live or end it.

I got help through the Fire Service Employee Assistance Program, which helped somewhat, but more because I felt such relief that I could speak to someone who listened. My subsequent CBT sessions did nothing to lift me from my depression.

This is when I was introduced to Caroline's Workshops through a colleague who again had been in a bad place. I didn't really know what to expect but mentally everywhere was dark, my head was in a fog and I couldn't really take anything in, so I was muddling through (the classic signs). During the Workshop, Caroline and Daniel taught me and the group a practice. To this day, I cannot believe the change. During my first session I just had an immense feeling of happiness, and from being so down I felt like I was smiling like the Cheshire Cat. During the second practice I relived a whole life of happy thoughts and visions. I couldn't have been in a happier place. Walking away from the Workshop was like walking from a dark room to brilliant light; the difference from the start to finish of the day. The subsequent days I could take things in again, I just felt 'if this is the life, I want some of this!' You never notice the small changes until it is too late and I hadn't realised I had ended up in that world.

I've carried on the practice for months and this has been the key to dealing with my issues. Things I struggled to talk about without breaking down now have closure on them. The images never go, but I can openly talk about the experience without issue.

This programme should be taught to all staff and new recruits as it's a tool that would save a lot of people such as myself, who endured a career of mental injuries that never manifest themselves until it's too late.

Military

One of the first veterans I worked with was in one of my early Workshops in Brighton. I remember him well; he came with his wife who shared with me she was supporting him as he had PTSD. He released something that day, although he hardly spoke. I questioned whether he got anything at all from the experience. It wasn't until 2018 that I would find out the answer to that question. I was blown away when he showed up at a Workshop; he had even kept the original support resources he received back in 2012! He had been keeping up the practice, but what was profound was that he was sociable and chatty, sharing his experiences and ideas. His PTSD was a thing of the past.

Mandy works with military veterans. We have had many clients attend due to her recommendation. There was one particular client who I will always remember. He attended a course at the studio. He never revealed he was ex-military. He was passing through and saw what I did and thought, 'Why not?'

We had a long chat and at the end of the course I asked him if he would be kind enough to write something of his experience that I could share. He said he would be happy to as one of his passions was writing! Here it is:

A Tale of Two Toms

I had been a long-serving soldier and since leaving the army had continued to work as a private security contractor in one conflict zone or another. My story is a very typical one: a few close shaves here and there, I had lost some good friends along the way, and had seen an unhealthy amount of human carnage.

Very typically, I believed I had taken it all in my stride. I signed up for it, earned some good money along the way and led what many would consider to be an interesting and varied life, so why should I complain?

But there was clearly a price to pay. In my case, recurring nightmares, heavy drinking, being highly irritable and perhaps the most damaging of all, a disturbing sense of guilt that hung over me like a dark cloud. I must stress this guilt was about nothing that I could specify. I had served with distinction in the military and had a sound reputation in civilian circles. I believed I had always operated in a moral and ethical manner, and prided myself on being the protector, not the assassin.

Was I suffering from PTSD? I didn't know, but as I pondered the question, I made a chance meeting with an old army buddy who had been officially diagnosed with it and had received counselling by the military. He told me of an incident which he believed had caused his PTSD. I had suffered numerous incidents of a similar nature, one which resulted in me being seriously injured.

Whatever was wrong with me, I felt I needed to resolve the issue, spurred on by the fact that I had broken up from yet another relationship. My drinking was getting out of hand, I couldn't get motivated about work and I could feel myself on a downward spiral. I had been in this dark place before, but I had always managed to keep it together and come out of it. But this time it was different, and I was conscious of the fact I really needed to talk to someone and, moreover, I needed some practical assistance.

Purely by chance, I came across TRE UK® on the internet. There was something about its simple approach that resonated with me. No re-living events, no long-term processes, no drugs, just a simple practice and you get a tool for life. It all seemed too good to be true. I'm a bit of a sceptic and not a believer in 'The Panacea', but the idea that the body and mind heal themselves if allowed to has always been a concept I could relate to.

I thought it would be madness not to give the TRE a try. So, a little apprehensive, I turned up at my first session with Caroline and I am so very glad I did!

Caroline is a no-nonsense sort of person and reminded me somehow of a kindly Sergeant Major I once served with. She is, to use a military term, Firm, Fair and Friendly. Translated, she was to the point, balanced in her view, and kind – the key attributes of a good leader and someone whom I immediately felt I could trust.

Perhaps the most poignant comment she made was that the development of TRE had involved the study of animal behaviour. She mentioned a zebra escaping from a lion and how it would stand and shake once it realised it had survived to graze another day. By chance (and there seemed to be a lot of chance events at this time in my life) I had witnessed that very same thing having just come back from a job in Africa. Suddenly the TRE made a lot of sense.

Clearly 'trembling' has some purpose and I also came to the realisation that to do so in my chosen profession was looked upon as a sign of weakness and to be avoided at all costs, particularly by leaders. However frightened one might be, 'the stiff upper lip' must be maintained and we must soldier on! OK, as a professional soldier I also realise the importance of this 'where the metal meets the meat', but what works for us as soldiers does not mean it will work for us for the rest of our lives.

So, what did TRE do for me? After the first session I noticed an immediate improvement in my ability to carry out day-to-day tasks. Everything used to seem like an uphill struggle and often the simplest set back would cause me to get extremely agitated. Not anymore.

Midway through the program, I began to look at people differently. Whilst I have never been a very tolerant person, now I could at least accept others' 'faults' and move on without getting upset myself. I also found I was cutting away from negative influences around me, but with no remorse or bad feeling.

By the end of the course, I was a different person. The old Tom was gone, along with the heavy drinking, nightmares and above all, that pervasive feeling of guilt. I believe it was this sense of guilt that was at the heart of the issue. Why the guilt? Who knows? Some suggest it's 'Survivor's Guilt', although it may also stem from something in my childhood, which was a very bumpy start in life to say the least.

The bottom line is I don't think it actually matters, and as our lives can become increasingly complex, perhaps one might never get to the root of the problem. What does matter is the feelings of guilt are no longer there, my life is back on track and several months on, even close friends have commented on how I've changed for the better. It is clear to me I have 'Sergeant Major' Purvey and TRE to thank for that!

Another client who was ex-SAS shared in a Workshop after a session: *I feel emotional, but I have not given into it as we have been trained not to.* I made it very clear that in the Workshop it was OK but when on his own he must let the emotions come. Now we know, it's official – they are TRAINED to suppress their emotions

This came to light when I had another veteran recommended by his psychologist. His girlfriend attended with him. She was a policewoman and although she had not planned to start the programme, she decided to support him by understanding more. Quite convinced she held no stress, the session was a revelation to her. He was quite reserved and reluctant to completely relax.

Before starting the second session a week later, she told me how on their way back home after their first session she cried her eyes out. She was releasing her 'date rape' and she spoke about it like she was talking about any ordinary, everyday experience. That is when you know you have healed from it, when you can talk about the trauma without the feelings and emotions.

It was during her partner's third session he whispered, 'I feel so angry.' I encouraged him to let it out. I am not sure I was ready for what happened, but he gave three raucous roars. I seriously thought the police would be knocking on the door to see who was being murdered! His psychotherapist got back to me after his session to say how noticeably less tense his face was.

It was this experience that highlighted for me just how much anger our military hold. No wonder that suppressed anger comes out in other ways, whether that is violence, anger, or the physical abuse of others. Such outbursts of anger have put many in prison.

Police

Someone close to me is in the Police, and I know how much they, like all others in the Service, give the 'I am OK' response. Thankfully, I have had clients from the Service; many have discovered the benefits, but are always reluctant to have that first 'conversation' with others! The big breakthrough came when a doctor who recommended a patient to us, seeing the TRE as a practical tool for the Police. Following a success in a small pilot Workshop, plans are now being made to extend to a wider cohort. We are excited to have the opportunity to change mindsets and who knows where it can lead!

As one officer, suffering anxiety, depression and had suicidal thoughts on more than one occasion, shared:

> *The upshot of doing one 20-minute session a week has meant that I have weaned myself off my depression medication which I have been on for nearly eight years. I am better able to counter my anxiety as well. I don't always do a session every week; sometimes when I feel the need, I may do two sessions but in general and I can't tell you why, it just works. Be open-minded, it could just change your life!*

Paramedics

Having worked with paramedics they are, understandably, the most challenged when it comes to trauma. Whilst they may not always be first on the scene, they most certainly have the ultimate responsibility in saving lives.

The first paramedic I worked with was someone I knew. She was curious and being off work for several months with anxiety, she started to do the course. Her biggest and most challenging trauma released in the first session. She soon found herself in a good place. When she returned to work, no one was interested in listening to what she had to say about the one thing that had the biggest impact on her well-being!

I have worked with other paramedics and most are really challenged with the Roller Coaster. They need a lot of support as they let go of the trauma.

There is still a lot of work to do changing mindsets. The prospect of the service sectors having a powerful self-help tool for instant release of the adrenaline and cortisol from their fight/flight after dealing with the trauma of others is a long-held vision. More and more now, I see it fast becoming a reality, for there is nothing that compares to the human body's own ability to heal.

> **'Facing up to things, working through them,
> that is what makes you strong.'**
>
> *Sarah Dessen*
> *Best-selling American novelist*

Caroline's Points to Ponder

1. If you are in or know someone in the service sector, can you relate to the shared issues of those you have read here?

2. Do you wear a 'painted smile'?

3. Do you see it in the eyes – yours or others?

*'As I walked out of the door
toward the gate
that would lead to my freedom,
I knew that if didn't leave my
bitterness and hatred behind,
I'd still be in prison.'*

Nelson Mandela
*Former President of South Africa, anti-apartheid revolutionary,
philanthropist and author of 'Long Walk to Freedom'*

Chapter Sixteen
...and Villains –
Setting Prisoners Free!

All who attended my early Events and Workshops would have heard my mantra 'Get me into prisons, they are full of angry children!' In 2016 I had a chance conversation with one of my yoga students who had learned to Release, who told me he worked in a prison and would put me in touch with someone. No sooner the word than the deed, it was not long before positive dialogue started. This was my first experience of feeling the frustration with the wheels of bureaucracy slowly turning, from prisons closing, to lack of funding and changing roles!

It was a great surprise when one morning in October 2017, I had an enthusiastic email asking me if I would like to go to teach yoga in the prison. I emailed back and explained that previous communications were not about yoga but something very different.

Daniel and I were invited to go and talk to those in charge of the prisoners' well-being. They were fascinated. Communications progressed, applications were processed and a couple of months later we returned for our induction and preparation for our first weekly visit on 3rd January 2018 to start a rolling six-week programme. This included other activities inmates engaged with on a daily basis such as arts, yoga, meditation and so on, for well-being.

Up bright and breezy, Daniel and I were parked up at the prison at 7.30 a.m. As we walked towards the gates, Daniel said to me, 'I feel a bit scared,' to which I replied, 'I am so excited – this is a dream come true!' We had no experience at all in this new world we were going to enter, but I was focused on our purpose. We were guided through the whole security process and with keys attached to our belts, I started to feel the intensity of prison life.

To support us on our first day, a member of the well-being team accompanied us to the room we were to be working in. Twelve inmates had signed up. This was indeed a pivotal day – for we did not know them, they did not know us. We had no technology to illustrate and deliver our message, just one shot to engage and intrigue – could we do this? I was first struck by their politeness. They walked in, respectfully called me 'Miss' and Daniel 'Sir', they shook hands and sat in the circle we had set up. I drew a deep breath and started to introduce who we were and what we were there for. They all engaged and went with the flow. An officer walked in towards the end as they were all lying on their side resting out. She said, 'I have never seen them so quiet, what have you done with them? And they would never turn their back to another inmate!'

The morning went better than I could have imagined. I have loved every session we have shared. We have also learned from every session, from that day on for over two and a half years, until Lockdown put us on pause!

Week on week, group after group shared their deepest fears, their hopes, their views and opinions about life in prison, politics, family, children and so much more.

Some of the things we learnt:

- Inmates are human beings – underneath there is a lost child.

- Drugs are a big problem – they are a get-by strategy.

- Some came to us with a mindset of hope for their future but some had none.

- Just like the service sector, they use laughter and jokes to mask their fears.

- They have some amazing insights and philosophies on life.

- They are stuck in more than just the physical prison – it's also their own physical, mental and emotional prison.

- For many, prison has been an 'interruption' to their life. They commit the crime, serve their time and then repeat the pattern.

- How to adapt our practice to really get them to engage.

- To speak their language in a way that has enabled us to keep returning.

- That we could walk through the grounds and would often be stopped by an inmate with a cheery smile who would be pleased to see us.

What inmates have learnt from us if they engage with a simple practice:

- They have a life tool and a tool for life.

- They have a Diamond that has yet to come out and shine.

- They can Release, to leave all their past behind so when they get out they not only find freedom from the walls of the prison, but freedom from their physical, mental and emotional prison.

- That by releasing anger, it moves away and they find inner peace. Free from their past.

- The need for drugs is no longer there.

- They are not 'triggered' by others.

- Their support network, both inside and outside the prison, comment on the positive changes.

We met young men who had gone through the Young Offenders system, gypsies (their terminology) inside with family members, men from different cultures, backgrounds and countries. And they all seemed to have something in common – a troubled childhood.

Snippets shared after sessions:

'I wish I had known this when I was eight, I would not be in here now.'

'For the first time I am asking myself "Who am I?" I have never done that before.'

'I could see that little boy in me, happy and carefree; it is like I have set him free.'

'I saw what my dad did to me, that was hard. I let it go.'

'I have never expressed emotion before this.'

'My pain has gone.'

'I felt burning in my leg – that is where I got shot.'

Carrying guilt

At the end of a session when all returned to the circle, the prisoners could share anything from their experience. One young man said he felt emotional, as he felt he had let his little sister down, when they were taken into care and he couldn't care for her. Tears started to flow. 'Look at me now, you all think I am a wuss.' But what followed was so touching. One by one every member of the circle got up, walked over to him and gave him a hug. The releasing was making them all more sensitive to others' needs, especially in the group. Before he left, I asked this young man how old he was when all this happened. He replied, 'Nine years old.' But for protocols, I would have given him a hug. I reminded him he was only a child then and it was neither his fault nor his responsibility. If he continues to Release and let go of the past, when he was free he would be a real support for his sister. It was all incredibly unexpected and profound to realise that he had held this anger into his thirties which most likely caused him inner pain and anger which then helped put him inside.

Reuniting with family

One week an inmate that had done the programme asked if he could share something with the group. He said, 'When I did a practice in the group, I saw myself as a baby and I saw my dad, though I have never met him! Recently I have now been in touch with him and learned I also have brothers. This programme has enabled me to reconnect with a family I never even knew I had!'

But I have dealt with it all!

We had started a new group and a seemingly confident young man, Paul, seemed really interested in our message. He was fascinated by his experience and said he was looking forward to the next week. But by then his tone had changed. He was 'politely' angry, saying how he had let go of his past, he had dealt with it and we had brought it all up. I let him share his reflections. I was then able to explain that this is exactly what our message is. We block and store in our body stuff that has never been dealt with in the past. By releasing and experiencing the feelings, emotions and memories, one is actually free, which is why we say 'Feel It to Heal It'!

Paul missed one of the six sessions. In the last session whilst all those in the group were releasing, he sat at a table with some card and pencils and was busy doing something. The group came together, and he asked them all to go over to join him. They sat down and shared their experience. Paul went last and said something which was so powerful, that today we share with all we teach. He said, 'I realised the worse I was feeling, the better I was getting.' He then handed over this card. On the front was he'd written:

> *Everybody wants Happiness*
> *Nobody wants Pain*
> *But you can't have a Rainbow*
> *Without a little Rain...*

I had never heard this before and was quite touched.

Inside he wrote:

> *Thank you both for everything you've done and continue to do. I hope with counselling and communication that one day I have half the positiveness you both have! You are both inspirational and pure souls. Thank you for emptying my Bucket!*

> *You are both very special and I along with the lads continue to talk about you and the powerful practice you do. Thank you for restoring my faith in others. Paul*

The card included many other endearing messages. One week a few months later, Paul came to find us. We sat for almost an hour having the best conversation. What a transformation! He called me when he was released, and he again shared his gratitude. It was great to know he had set himself free in more ways than one!

The story of Marcus

We met Marcus, a nice-looking young man who had only just turned 30. Smartly dressed and polite, but clearly on drugs. After his first session he was sobbing so I sat with him a while. He told me he had lost everything and had nothing to live for. He had lost both his parents, his aunt and uncle, and his baby daughter whose name was tattooed on his arm. All he had left was his sister. I reassured him that if he had a sister, then he certainly did have something to live for. Marcus really connected with the practice; we saw the best of him and the worst of him and he came and went and at one point even disappeared for a while. One day he reappeared, a new man. We shared many a good conversation and Marcus became an ambassador for our work. I asked him one day if he would like to share his story, for he certainly had one to tell. I had only heard bits, but when he started to share what happened in his childhood, it all fell into place. I think it sums up the reason why many men and women end up in prison and youngsters end up in Young Offenders Institutions.

> *Up to the age of 11, my life seemed idyllic. I had a pleasant childhood with parents who loved me. At school I stood out in sports, particularly football.*

I was so good I was sent to an academy with 50 other kids from Kent. Only 10 could go through, and I was one of those 10. All this promise dissipated when my mum died of alcohol poisoning. I suddenly found myself in care, separated from my sister and being shunted from foster home to foster home. I was expelled from school, but my reprieve came a few years later when my sister became old enough to become my legal guardian.

By the age of 15, I started messing about with soft drugs and was jailed for the first time. Both sets of grandparents died and my drug use escalated to harder substances. I had a bad motorbike accident, breaking my femur in seven places as well as breaking my arm. After leaving hospital, I spent several months in a wheelchair and on crutches.

At the age of 22, my auntie and uncle died. I did not feel a sense of loss because I was harbouring resentment for the fact that the family home (which had been left to me and my sister) had been stolen by them on Mum's death. They were also responsible for putting us into care.

At 26 I received a call from my sister telling me to get over to Dad's flat as soon as possible. I found him face down on the bathroom floor, dead from alcohol poisoning. He had been there for three days…

I was 26 years old with no Mum and Dad, no grandparents, aunties and uncles. I continued self-medicating with hard drugs but somehow managed to find a nice girl. She was a prison officer and we planned to have children together. At 26 weeks into the pregnancy, she lost the baby which traumatised us both greatly. My drug use again escalated as I struggled to cope.

My life continued to spiral out of control until I received a five-year prison sentence aged 30. Two years into the term, I found myself in a drug-induced coma, cuffed to a hospital bed for two months. The coma was so bad, they played music to keep me alive. They thought I would have to be in a wheelchair and the mad house for the rest of my days. Upon regaining consciousness, I could not articulate myself properly. I was so delusional, I thought I could bite through the cuffs and lost several teeth in the process. I had to wear a spit and bite mask as my behaviour was so bad. I was laying in my own piss and shit on a prison hospital bed. I could not remember my family or friends.

Once I returned to jail, I dropped from 16 stone to 10 and felt so hopeless. But despite this desperate situation, one thing that did keep coming into my head was when someone in the same cell as me died. That did not help my mental health. I tried to hang myself. I was hallucinating, but then I saw my parents and unborn little girl looking down upon me and I no longer wanted to die as I felt they wanted me to live.

I started doing a course in jail called 'See Life More Clearly'. Part of this included a module called the Total Release Experience®, taught by Caroline and Daniel from outside. During the first session I found myself crying with a profound sense of release and relief. The second session found me crying again. What I noticed was that all my trauma from my life and the deaths of my family were coming up. But Caroline explained to me that things would seem to get worse before they got better and boy, was she right! I started releasing from my bucket twice a week because of the pressure of dealing with life in the prison.

I was releasing from 'outside' problems; it was helping the pain from the pins and plates in my leg from the motorbike accident years before. It was helping the nerve damage in both hands, plus overcoming the terrible drug-induced coma.

I was diagnosed with Personality Disorder (PD)* plus I suffered Post-Traumatic Stress Disorder (PTSD). When I tried hanging myself, I did not want to die but I just could not articulate what I needed to say.

I was still not myself but got back onto the Total Release Experience® course. I started to realise that I am a Diamond – I had just lost my shine and was now getting a polish! Plus, without the practice of releasing from my bucket, it would fill back up a lot quicker around others in prison. But the day I got back on the mat and started releasing with the best people in the world, things just got better.

Every time I get down on that mat, no matter how bad a day I have had or how bad my mental health is affecting me, I always get up a new man.

---

* See glossary at the back for the full meaning.

I've done this for eight months now and it's cleared all my injuries, helped me with my addictions and so much more. Yes, I am going to say I wasted 12 years of my life in prison, but this Release Experience is giving me a different way of life that allows me to cope with challenges. I get on my mat and Release negative emotions to keep them from going in my bucket. I keep my bucket empty by doing 20 minutes laying on my mat, once or twice a week.

It's truly amazing opening myself up by releasing. I believe in what Caroline and Daniel are doing. They are so caring, and I am not the only prisoner to benefit as they help anyone who wants to learn and is troubled. I would like to say thank you to both of them. I mean that from the bottom of my heart. It's been an emotional roller coaster as I continue to deal with my past to this day because you don't empty your bucket overnight.

It has been life-changing for me and is still changing my life for the better. Now I have no pains of old injuries, no back ache or headaches. I feel more confident and I feel I can handle the pressures outside of prison, with bills and day-to-day life. I am coping with drug addiction a lot better. I am more and more mindful about my thought processes, especially with my mental health. I feel so healthy that my Diamond is really shining, and people notice that day to day. I just have that glow about me. I was a nervous wreck before but now with so much confidence. Thank you, you changed my life.

Today I am thinking about my actions and a lot more aware of my body. I am just thinking so much clearer, not just about my exterior but my interior. This programme is an amazing part of my life. Without it, I don't think I could have bounced back so quickly, just three to four months after people were convinced I was going to die. If the Total Release Experience® Programme had not worked for me, I would still be in that old black hole.

When I am released from prison, how will I feel in the next year as I deal with day-to-day life and how will I get on with my drug addictions?

When I read this, and even as I write it up, I come back to my raison d'être – get me into prison as it is full of angry children! This story pulls the whole message together. That from one generation to another, trauma is passed on; mum and dad masking their problems with self-medication, how a child can so easily go off the rails and how then one thing leads to another. My heart skips a beat reading this story as there are thousands of stories out there that will NEVER get told, for they have buckets so full but no way to Release them. How many will end up taking their own life? How many will be assumed to be the low life of the earth because of their drugs problem? How many will serve their time, but only reoffend and return to prison?

When I heard the then Prison Minister Rory Stewart saying that he was investing in the prison service, and if the anger and the drugs were not sorted out before the end of the year he would resign, I laughed and said out loud, 'You might as well go now, for if you believe £80 million is going to solve the problem, forget it!' No amount of sniffer dogs or officers is going to HEAL the cause. For the cause is stuck in buckets that they cannot access. Imagine the savings for the Service if all the inmates got to learn to Release! If they could step outside the gates free of their past like Marcus, families would be happier, society would be safer, reoffending would be highly unlikely, and the prospect of a new life would be greater.

Marcus is Free now; I hope when he is ready, he will get in touch and share his Part Two!

Many officers, including those who mentored the inmates we worked with, would stop us as we walked through and remark on the transformations they had noticed.

One female officer came to me and said, 'I have been off for six weeks with stress and anxiety. When do officers get to attend the programme? It is not fair that they [the inmates] get it and we don't.'

I replied, 'When your Seniors value the importance of your well-being.' That officer stood her ground in a staff meeting and raised the question. From that we were due to start with the officers just after Lockdown! One day soon, it will happen. I have a vision that prisons will become unrecognisable!

**'Education is the most powerful weapon
which you can use to change the world.'**

Nelson Mandela
*Former President of South Africa, anti-apartheid revolutionary,
philanthropist and author of 'Long Walk to Freedom'*

Caroline's Points to Ponder

1. Do you know someone in prison? What do you know about their childhood?

2. Have you ever been in Young Offenders or prison? Can you resonate with any of Marcus' story?

3. Having read Paul and Marcus' stories, what view do you have now about inmates?

'Beautiful are those whose
brokenness gives birth
to transformation and wisdom.'

John Mark Green,
Australian thriller writer and publisher

Chapter Seventeen
Set Yourself Free –
Shine Bright Like A Diamond

We teach everyone how transformational the practice can be; that with regularity, you heal from your past, you build resilience, but more importantly, you are set free, layer by layer and can transform your life.

It makes sense that as you peel away, layer by layer, the negative energy from your body clears. The Diamond gets a little polish with every session so it then shines through more and more.

Clients' life-changing decisions include getting back with their partner, leaving their partner, changing job or career, moving house and even migrating to another country. Fulfilling dreams they never dared to dream! On another level, many have reconnected with the arts, such as singing, painting, playing guitar or piano. That in itself is wonderful. Being able to speak out, having found their voice, been given the confidence to say what they want, to be able to stand up and say NO when they want to. Men and women transform their lives by finally knowing what it is they want for themselves and go after it. Here are two more stories of people who have done just that!

Nessie – A Diamond like no other

Nessie originally joined one of my yoga classes in the autumn of 2013 and decided to try the TRE in the New Year.

She had been stuck in a cycle of self-destructive behaviour since the age of 15 (she was now 33). She initially struggling with anorexia, moving into bulimia and self-harming, to compulsive shopping and finally, online gambling.

Her history is complicated. Her dad has suffered mental health problems most of her life and so she was a withdrawn and compliant child and an easy target. The main trauma was being targeted by a gang of boys at secondary school. She was sexually assaulted nearly every day at school for three years, including being gang raped on no less than four occasions. But sexual bullying is such a taboo subject that the school branded her 'hypersensitive' and unable to cope with it emotionally, and her father disowned her. Whilst the sexual assaults came to light while she was at school, she wasn't able to talk of the gang rapes until aged 31. This was compounded by losing her gran to cancer at the age of 15 and her dad suffering a heart attack and cardiac arrest two weeks before her 17th birthday. She felt like she was being punished for what had happened.

She felt like she had been on a mission to prove everyone wrong, from those who branded her hypersensitive, and those who said she would never get a qualification, to those who said she would never hold a job down. Whilst her personal life had been nearly non-existent, she managed a successful career but felt she was going through the motions of daily life, not really living: stuck in a bubble, unable to reach out and connect with anyone. From the age of 15, she had been in different talking therapies and tried antidepressants on several occasions, which just made her symptoms worse. Despite some change with the support of counselling and EMDR, she felt the TRE has helped her take another step forward; to reconnect with her body and find her voice.

Nessie takes up her story: *I used to be physically unable to move and often unable to speak when experiencing flashbacks. I am calmer and less overwhelmed on a day-to-day basis and my sleep pattern has improved. I feel more alert and more able to connect and interact with people. The TRE is like waking up and coming out of a fog; the world seems brighter.*

Having used compulsive shopping and online gambling as coping mechanisms, I had amounted debts in excess of £12,000 but I cleared the debts in 18 months without assistance and accumulated savings. A high point was owning my car outright, but more significantly, at 39 years old I was able to begin living independently for the first time and enjoy the freedom of debt-free living. In addition to the compulsive shopping, I collected and hoarded but step by step I released all my collections and now live a very minimalist life. I felt so ashamed of my life then but now I can hold my head high and feel proud that I turned it around.

After having withdrawn from all activities apart from work for over 10 years, I undertook a year-long Personal Embodiment training course involving movement, drawing and creative writing. Having never driven more than 50 miles from my home, I drove over 200 miles to attend and stayed away from home for the first time.

My creativity has always been important to me but I never believed my work was of a good enough standard; but to date I have had three poems published in two anthologies.

Physically I have pushed through barriers and beliefs. Having joint hypermobility and patella realignment surgery at 27, I was told I would never be able to run and yet I can now run! I've had to address a lot of phobias in relation to food, but in the last six months, I have been able to adopt a much healthier diet. I have now lost a stone in weight and am no longer considered overweight for my height.

I have been able to make changes in my career, but I know the best is yet to come and I have plans to walk away from my 21-year public sector career by the end of the year. I don't know where that will lead me, but I know something better waits for me.

What I really want to say is that I thought things could never get better and that I was an unfixable freak. More than anything, I wanted validation of my experiences and the most important learning for me was learning that my body keeps the score, my body remembers, and that is all the validation I need.

I will always feel connected to Nessie and be ever grateful that she put her trust in me. She taught me so much about the power of the human body to heal, and that was priceless learning. It was a privilege to be able to work together through each session until she felt strong enough to practice on her own. It was in one particular session we looked at each other as I checked in on her experience and she laughed. We both laughed, for finally, like no other session before, all seemed OK. Not the end, but a turning point. I am so proud of what she has achieved for herself. From the introverted, frightened young lady with no hope for her future and no self-esteem, she stepped up and took control. I am as excited for her now about her future as she is for herself.

Darren – rediscovered his true self

I met Darren many years ago on a yoga training programme. We connected on and off over the years, and then he started to teach a weekly early morning yoga class at my Centre. He was in his early forties with two young boys; he worked full time on his father's farm. He had been doing this for as long as he could remember. He was also a freelance swimming teacher and much in demand. My own grandson had lessons with him. He is great with children and knew his craft.

When I started with the TRE, Darren would always say he never saw the need for it as he did yoga and swimming and life was good. It was something he often reminded me of over the first six years of my evolving journey.

To my surprise, it was Mother's Day in 2017, and Darren said he wanted to pay for a friend to attend a Workshop. The friend was a social worker, and Darren knew him to be suffering with anxiety and other symptoms of stress. Darren thought he would support his friend and so attend with him, possibly just to satisfy his own curiosity too, which I guess had come from years of me 'batting on' about what it was doing for others. They both left feeling different.

I met Darren after his early morning yoga class, as I did every so often, to take him for breakfast so we could have a catch-up. He started to share his experiences with the releasing he was doing with regularity. 'You know, I thought my peripheral vision was out here,' he gestured his arms out, 'Now it is here,' and widened them as far as he could reach. He shared that he had come to be awakened on many levels. One particular realisation was his position within his direct family; as the youngest child of three, the reality that he was never taken seriously, and at times ridiculed featured more strongly now than before his releasing experience. He said, 'Releasing has helped me to understand, and wake up to the fact, that the life I've lived on the farm isn't the one I wish to pursue. Over recent years my ethics have changed, and they no longer match that of a traditional beef farm. I have been living the life my dad wanted me to; a change had to happen, it was going to be painful, but ultimately necessary, and right for me and my family.'

Every time we met it was always the same: not five minutes would pass, and then he would talk passionately about the power of his releasing, and the sharing stories. Darren often felt overworked and rarely had time to relax. He made the decision to give up his role as a swimming teacher, a position he had held for nearly 20 years, although he still had plenty to keep him busy, what with supporting his wife with her Forest School, as well as yoga and the farm.

He was often in awe of what was going on in my world and how my journey was evolving and ever changing. He attended a second Workshop in 2018 with his wife who wanted to learn. He had also shown his young boys who were curious when they saw him early morning laying on the floor releasing. Sharing with little ones is something we actively encourage.

One morning we were sat outside for another breakfast catch-up in the sunshine and he shared something that made my jaw drop. He had decided with his wife to convert a big van, sell their house, take their boys out of school and leave the UK to have an adventure. Wow, I was not expecting that! Whilst I immediately realised I would be losing a much-loved friend and yoga teacher, it was just fantastic to see that together, as a family, they had a dream, and were going for it. Truly transformational!

One morning in September 2019, we met outside the yoga centre to say our goodbyes. The way he had created a home on four wheels was amazing. They were well aware, however, that space would be limited and that may well bring challenges, but they all knew they had something that took up no room in their space – their ability to maintain optimum well-being and build resilience. They had their Total Release Experience®. It was to serve them well!

In March 2020 Lockdown was beginning to impact the world; and as beautiful as the view was in Portugal, parked opposite a lake, a decision had to be made before the borders closed. They drove back to the UK. On Friday 12th June at 7.30 a.m. I set off to meet Darren on Dover seafront. It was great to see him. We sat two metres apart in his mobile home and shared coffee. After 30 minutes of hearing the highlights of the trip and a general catch-up, we spent three hours sharing stories about the release experience! There were times that if they had not had the knowledge and tools to be able to Release, the consequences could have been disastrous! The great thing is they did it – all of them – even the children. They are one special family. The perfect parenting tool and the perfect family survival tool!

'Don't let your history interfere with your destiny.'

Steve Maraboli
Motivational speaker, behavioural scientist and
best-selling author of 'Life, the Truth and Being Free'

Caroline's Points to Ponder

1. What has been the most transformational experience you have had?

2. Do you dare to dream? What would living your dream look like?

3. Was there ever a time you felt so low you did not want to live? What stopped you?

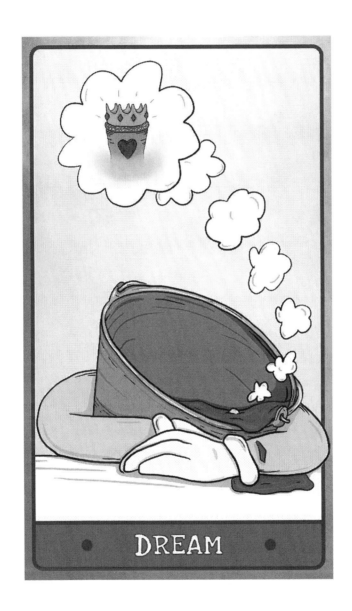

DREAM

'Love yourself...
enough to take the actions
required for your happiness...
enough to cut yourself loose
from the drama-filled past...
enough to move on.'

Dr Steve Maraboli
Motivational speaker, behavioural scientist and
best-selling author of 'Life, the Truth and Being Free'

Chapter Eighteen
Finding Your Truth –
Mary's Journey

You have read some incredible insights as to the power of the body to heal itself. I have one more to share with you which makes it very clear that if you want change, if you want to set yourself free, you have to do it **yourself.** There is no timescale, there is no 'sneak peak' at what is releasing next, but whatever your body releases it is your body, your History and only yours to Release. Whatever comes up, you have to keep going; you will finally get to the TRUTH about how you came to be the person you are today. When you find the truth, you finally set yourself free.

Mary's is a story of just how tough the journey can be. She is determined to find her Truth, and despite her dark and scary journey, she is never giving up.

Mary – a Woman of Courage

It was March 2017 when Mary called. She was distraught for she had seen TRE exercises on YouTube and tried to emulate them but in the process had re-traumatised herself. She was upset because she felt 'that even if I could get on the floor to do the exercises for the tremoring, there was no space to do it.'

I was able to reassure her that everything could be adapted to suit her. Mary was very challenged and was seeking yet (another) way to try and heal. She was a victim of a narcissistic/sadistic mother and an emotionally weak and violent father; 'toxic parents', as she would call them. I warmed to Mary straight away as she was clearly an articulate and intelligent woman. She was morbidly obese and a self-confessed hoarder. It was not long before we started to work together on Skype. We soon got around the limitations and as she lay on her bed she started her first Release experience. She said afterwards, 'Oh my God, this is amazing. This is nothing like what I was doing via YouTube!'

Mary reminded me, 'If it hadn't been for you saying to me, "Don't worry about that! We can adapt to the exercises; we can adapt everything," I could never have done it.'

Mary's healing journey was never going to be easy, but at least she was on it. We had been working together regularly for a few weeks when Daniel moved to the UK. I shared Mary's story with him and said I really wanted to support her back to 'being Mary'. Daniel took over her sessions. He loved working with Mary and every week he would delight in reporting back to me the impact the sessions were having on her. I was there to mentor and advise. They found it easy to connect and to talk; he was just what Mary needed. Mary's challenges have been phenomenal, her story is a book in itself.

There were some big shifts for Mary fairly early in July 2017 She became vegan – something she always wanted to do but had never been able to.

She had a dream she shared with Daniel, that she wanted to live by the sea in Herne Bay and was taken aback when Daniel said, 'Why don't we meet up in Herne Bay and I can show you around, because that's where I was born!' She couldn't believe it. But at that time, she was so overwhelmed as she had a fear of men, people, and going out in general, that she felt really stressed out by it so could not do it.

In August 2017, Mary shared another significant moment.

> *I walked past a mirror in my flat and briefly glanced into it. This is something I usually avoid doing at all costs because for the whole of my life, whenever I*

peer into a mirror all I ever see is my mother staring back at me with her cold, sinister, angry, disapproving eyes. Ever since I disassociated as a very young child, I feel possessed by my mother and I have never seen myself, EVER but THIS TIME staring back at me was…me. I was overcome with grief and sobbing for the loss of me interspersed with wonderful feelings of giddiness as if I had just locked eyes with the love of my life. In that moment…looking at my own eyes, looking straight back at me with kindness and gentleness… I realised that I had been brainwashed by my narcissistic mother.

Remember that dream of going to Herne Bay? Mary planned a holiday in Kent with her mother in 2018. Daniel again suggested they meet in Herne Bay – and this time they did! It was completely significant for Mary because not only did she get out, but she went on holiday and met a man!

Mary says: *Releasing is the greatest adventure of my life. But it's also the most painful thing of my life. I'm not going to stop, no matter how bad it gets. Because I so much want to be free. I want to experience peace within myself. I've always had this thing within me, that there is a cure. But I have tried all sorts to find that cure, and at last I now believe I have it. I want to be free.*

I get very pessimistic about that, only because everything is getting so intense. I feel things are really shifting, it is horrible, I feel I am at the coalface now, going into a very dark place at the moment, very, very dark. What is coming up now I've never felt before because this is the stuff that I did a massively wonderful job of suppressing. I've never felt this but I'm not going to give up, never.

I want to be free, I want to know what it's like to love. And that's another part of me that I'm realising. Many things have been coming up recently that have given me a massive insight into what my mother did. She completely destroyed every natural instinct in me and what I mean by that, is the natural instinct to be feminine. The natural instinct to love and to be loved. The natural instinct to be myself. The natural instinct to be human, basic core stuff, she completely destroyed within me. I'm actually discovering things about humanity that I didn't even know existed.

I used to say to Daniel, "Do you know what is going to happen next? How much longer is it going to go on for?" He would say, "No one knows, for it is not my story but your story. We are all on our own journey, you know, and what's going to happen to you is not what's going to happen to me. You are on a unique journey back to yourself."

What is happening to Mary now is real. It is amazing that she is at last getting to the truth, the truth of her trauma. The truth of what happened to her. The truth that she always thought was within her but because she never had the support, she could never look inwards and unlock it. Now she has the key to unlock the truth and as she releases, something leaves, getting her closer to the truth. All that has been said to her – the meanness and humiliation–– to her, it is alive. By regressing back to childhood, she is literally witnessing the truth, as it is revealing what is inside of her, and what really happened to her.

She has felt enormous distress and abandonment, but then it is suddenly released. Mary says: *It was lovely. I felt relief, and then all of a sudden, I could see inside myself. I could see what arises, what the next feeling would be. I could see it because emotions are energy in motion.*

When challenged with holding a lifetime of trauma in the body, the roller coaster seems to go on and on. Mary has had many, many ups and downs. We know, as Mary does, that she is still peeling away the layers. What we love about Mary, is how different she is in herself; she continues to have a weekly session with Daniel, and he is always there to support her, as I am. Mary's life hit her hard and left its mark, but she is slowly, layer by layer, emptying her bucket. She continues to inspire us with her courage, bravery, and determination to keep going. She loves and believes in the power of the practice and our philosophy. She is getting stronger and has different transformations as she continues to deal with the trauma of her past and other life challenges.

We love Mary and will be there for her always. Her story is testimony that not all have the 'instant' miracle, but she is a Diamond like no other and we notice the sparkle that glimmers through every so often. She is going to shine like no other. Many would have given up by now, but not Mary.

She is giving herself enough love to drive through this incredible journey of hers, finally getting to the truth where she will then be free.

> **'Freedom means the opportunity to be**
> **what we never thought you would be.'**
>
> *Daniel J Boorstin*
> *American historian and award-winning author*

Caroline's Points to Ponder

1. Have you ever found something so hard that you gave up on it?

2. What do you see when you look in the mirror?

3. Do you know your Truth?

*'If you think you are too small
to make a difference,
you haven't spent the night
with a mosquito.'*

African proverb

Chapter Nineteen
Malawi – Leaving a Footprint

In September 2018 Daniel came out of his online meeting and said, 'Ania, a successful Confidence Coach in my Accountability group, is organising an expedition to Malawi. She just asked the group if we knew an entrepreneurial woman who would like to join, as someone had to drop out. I told her I did – she will be sending you an email!'

Malawi? I didn't even know where it was other than in Africa. The BBC had been sharing the story of the kidnapped schoolgirls, and I knew it was one of the poorest countries in the world. I had hardly got to ask Daniel a question and the email came through. I read:

The Purpose of this Expedition:

is to bring women together who are passionate about leaving an impactful footprint in this world. Women who want to be challenged, pushed out of their comfort zone, share skills and expertise, learn from new cultures, grow new collaborations and networks, to inspire hope for tomorrow. Women who also want to hit the pause button in the beauty of Africa, to redefine their business and personal goals

The Challenge:

Climbing Mount Mulanje (Malawi's highest mountain in southern Malawi).

I was shopping when my telephone rang – it was Ania. We had never met, but straight away I felt a connection; I think we both did. I went back to my car while she told me about her mission. She and her family had been impacted by seven suicides and she wanted to put something back into life and make a difference. I shared with her my work and we did not stop talking. She said, 'Look, it is a lot to take in. I know it is short notice as we go in five weeks, but think about it.' Straight away I said, 'I don't need to, I am going!' I just thought if I could share what I do to change lives, I would. It was also the opportunity of a lifetime. We were both emotional. I dashed home, made a cup of coffee, and said to my husband and Daniel, 'In the garden, we are having a meeting!' Somewhat surprised and probably wondering what was so important, we sat down, and I announced, 'On 13th October I am going on an expedition to Malawi.' The look of surprise was an absolute picture! I quickly explained my conversation with Ania and then knowing they were both right behind me, I got into gear and started to plan. I was going to need about £3.5k for this trip with flights and everything else, money I didn't have!

Needs must, I did something I have never done – fundraise! I set up a GoFundMe page and emailed all my TRE UK® clients and yoga students as well as any others I could think of. The response was amazing; from such kindness and generosity, I raised £1.7k. Beautiful messages such as:

- I hope it does for them what it has done for me.

- I believe in the practice of the TRE for healing and change, and wish to support spreading it to others far and wide and to support others who have the passion to do just that.

- Go, Caroline! Your work is life enhancing and miraculous.

- So inspiring to hear you supporting so many women, and prisoners, good on ya!

- A great cause, they'll benefit from your knowledge as I have :)

- I have benefited greatly from the TRE so want you to help other people. Good luck!

What was interesting about the whole preparation experience were the reactions. There were plenty that were so excited for me, as well as those that thought I was mad! At my age, going off and doing all on the agenda and a challenge to climb Mount Mulanje! One of my yoga students asked in class if I was worried about the mountain challenge. Another responded and said, 'You can do that, you are a yoga teacher!' I replied, 'Of course – it is just one foot in front of the other, isn't it!'

Famous last words…!

I was all set to go but needed walking boots for the mountain climb. I happened to be working in Swindon so stayed with my special niece, always so supportive of what I was doing. I was so chuffed to leave with her boots in my car – the perfect fit. All set to go!

Malawi, here we come

On 13th October I arrived at Heathrow, having stopped on the way to connect with each of my children. Although they were all proud, I think there was a little bit of apprehension, but they know their mother!

I had already met most of the group as we had a meeting in London which was not just an opportunity to meet each other, but to all be interviewed for a radio show, and when we were given our T-shirts, which was great for spotting each other at the airport. The camaraderie was fantastic.

Before we knew it, we were up in the air and on our way. It was a very long trip – almost 19 hours. We landed at Blantyre airport, which was exceedingly small. It took a while to get checked through. We first had to exchange money – can you imagine almost 1,000 Kwacha to the Pound Sterling!

Lots of willing smiling faces came to greet us and wanting to take our bags to the bus that was awaiting us, and what an art their packing was! All aboard and Ron introduced himself, as did Justin, our driver; they were going to be looking after us throughout the trip. They were two men that I immediately felt safe with; in fact, we all did.

Settling in but not for long!

After a long journey, we settled into Fisherman's Rest. On Saturday evening, we enjoyed a meal in the garden, and all got to connect as Ania shared the week's busy programme. Zina suggested going to church the next morning, so on Sunday morning those of us that chose to go set off. That was a service and a half! Packed full of worshippers. I just loved listening to gospel singing. The messages and preaching were very profound. Our hearts melted.

We then all regrouped and travelled to various locations to attend our chosen meeting: HIV/Aids, Radio, Women's Rights and Mental Health, which was my choice. It was absolutely amazing to listen to what stresses, anxieties and traumas the Malawian people have to deal with, as well as making real connections and being able to share stories.

My first ambassador

Time was very tight. When the meeting finished and we'd had refreshments, I asked the young policeman Chiyemkezo if there was anyone he thought might like to connect with my work. He immediately responded and said, 'I would!' I could not believe it! The universe again was listening. This was his only day off and we were on the move the next day so we arranged that he came to our afternoon location and I would break away from the group and work with him. Later that afternoon as the clock ticked, I wondered whether he meant it; he had no car so would have to take a taxi. But right on time, there he was. I had already asked Ron if I could have cloth for the ground.

I gave Chiyemkezo an overview using image cards I had. He lay on the ground and was just starting to tremor when the sun disappeared, and spots of rain started to fall. Just what was needed! We picked up our things and ran over to a corrugated roof shelter where cars were parked. Without fuss, he got on the ground with only the cloth between him and concrete. Again, he started to Release. Not for long though, as the heavens opened. We had no choice but to run for shelter into the group's space. We walked through to the bottom end of the room and I asked

Ron if we could use the floor space between the desks. No problem! Chiyemkezo lay on the floor and before long he was releasing again. This went on for about 20 minutes. When he sat up, he had the biggest smile. After our chat, the group discussion had finished, and I introduced him as TRE UK®'s first Malawian Ambassador and I was going to train him to teach! He got a big round of applause. He travelled on the bus with us back to our lodging and I gave him a set of image boards. We exchanged details, I gave him back his taxi fare and Ron dropped him off on his way home. It could not have worked out any better!

I was elated as you might imagine. Chiyemkezo, with his Chief's blessing, would be sharing the Total Release Experience® with those in Malawi he worked with. He is also a safeguarding school officer too and was very excited about the work and those he could reach.

Trinitas – an inspirational woman

We went to Trinitas' workplace – she had been at the meeting the day before. What an inspiration! She makes washable sanitary wear; the biggest problem for girls is not being able to attend school when they have a period, as they have no money for sanitary wear. She told us her inspirational story of how she suffered herself as a girl and decided to do something about it. She took big chances and now is slowly building something amazing, with limited resources.

She has a lovely man that helps her to cut patterns and sew the products. She travels to South Africa twice a year to get the best materials, so that her product is absorbent and hygienic. She presents them in a pack of seven, although sold as single items. Genius idea! I think there is a lot of scope here; the savings would be phenomenal and teenage girls would not have to miss school.

Quality was the overriding factor for Trinitas. Although she has competition offering something cheaper, the risks to end users is greater. She sticks to her values and principals. I love that – a women unto my own heart. She was expecting her first baby in December after many previous complications.

Samaritans

After a photo call, we left Fisherman's Rest to go to the Samaritans Centre, located near to the orphanage from where Madonna adopted her children. Stella gave us a talk about all the good work they do to inspire children and teenagers, empowering them to be inspired, giving them hope to create a better future for themselves. I was able to donate some of the things for children I bought with the funds I had raised.

Stella shared the plight of children, many of whom are often abandoned by parents. When parents split up – maybe because the mother was abused – she then struggles to feed her family and so abandons her children. It is the wonderful work of those such as Stella that keeps the children going, to alleviate their stress and anxiety from their traumas.

We then set off, stopped for lunch and I spotted two zebras together –special! We visited a tea plantation before driving to the base camp, as tomorrow we would climb Mount Mulanje!

I did not see this coming

Arriving at the base camp, we settled into our lodges. I shared with two others. Unfortunately, after supper I had an accident and banged my head on a low-level tap in the shower! Sam was a nurse and stopped the bleeding and Fiona was there with her oils. I slept well and was up at 4.00 a.m. to prepare for the climb. Ania had asked me if I would share my work at the top of the mountain! We were to go for breakfast for 5.00 a.m. but by 4.30 I was sick – great! I was told there would be no mountain climb for me! I was to go and get checked out. I was mortified. I went back for a sleep and after the others had set off, Ron took me to a clinic to see a doctor.

Wow, we have no idea how lucky we are here in the UK…

It was basic beyond belief! The female doctor was very kind but had to find a scrap of paper to write on, before guiding me to the next room. I sat on a blood-stained sheet on a couch. Plugs were hanging off the wall and the door handle was falling off. She did a malaria test and all was clear. She said I needed stitches. Having never had stitches in my life, this was surreal! I questioned her to be sure – this was not just about money. We moved to another room, and had the suture pack not come out of a sterile pack, there is no way I would have stayed! Despite my concerns, I left there with two neat stitches in my head and something to stop the nausea – which was (fortunately) totally unrelated. I remembered that we had stopped for lunch on the way to the tea plantation. It was a hot day and I had forgotten the rules and ate a salad washed in their water! Just pure coincidence!

Step up or give up!

Back on the bus at 9.00 a.m., Ron asked me what I would like to do. Go back for a rest, or go and see some sights. I said, 'Ron, I want to climb the mountain!' My only thoughts were that I had come all this way to complete a challenge and that was important. How could I go back to the UK and say I couldn't do it because of feeling sick and had a couple of stitches in my head?! More to the point, how could I tell my niece her boots never made it up the mountain?!

The group organiser was busy sending messages, trying to persuade me not to go because of the heat and what would happen if I fell ill up the mountain.

I asked Ron not to take the call, and was it possible or was I mad? He said, 'I know you; you are a strong woman. Yes, it is possible!' He made a phone call and said, 'I am going to take you back so you can prepare and then we will meet our guides at the base camp.' We picked up David, the climb's organiser, on the way.

By 10.00 a.m., I was ready to go! I paid for two young male guides who were amazing. Still feeling sick, having not eaten anything, up since 4.00 a.m. and feeling like I had no energy, we set off. One step in front of the other, literally – I thought of those words I had shared with my yoga students! I was indeed going to be challenged. The guides said we were going to take a different route to the others. Instead of walking up the side, we were going straight up, and it was incredibly steep – well, it was 3,002 metres! I kept stopping and sometimes almost crawling up. My breath was my fuel, just as I tell my students! Every time we stopped, the guides gave me water and took pictures for me as I could not hold my camera. They knew the mountain like the back of their hand.

Don't ask me how, but after just over four hours, I finally made it. I could not believe it either when the guide said, 'You have arrived before the others; I can see them coming along the path!' I don't know who was more pleased, but they were just blown away to see me. The TRE I do for myself was indeed a test of my resilience. The Universe decided I should be challenged – I most definitely was. I had raised my bar and kept going, no matter how difficult things seemed to be.

We finally arrived at the lodge, which was just like something from *The Waltons* TV show – and after a short sleep, I felt more human. We had a great evening; we ate, laughed, and sang. I shared a TRE session with everyone, including George, the Chief Mountain Guide. He was blown away too. So now I had my second recruit! By 9.00 p.m., lights were out. It was challenging to get much sleep in a small room of 14 people. There was a lot of shuffling and moving around.

At 4.00 a.m. we were up and with four others who were physically challenged, we set off an hour ahead to go down the longer route. I was delighted that I would get to see and experience both aspects of the mountain. The second group went down the way I came up! They said to me, 'How on earth did you do that climb?' How on earth indeed!

The whole experience was nothing short of amazing. Once down – a shower was never more welcome – we said goodbye to the good guys and set off to a hotel for a treat.

Destiny I call it!

The next day was REALLY special. We went to the YODEP Children's Centre where we were greeted by cheering children, drums playing and adults swaying. We could feel the warmth of the welcome. Everyone gathered and introductions were made as the YODEP leaders spoke of the work they do. There are so many problems for the children they care for: mental health issues, discrimination, disabilities, poverty, abuse, abandonment and HIV. One could not help but be in awe of the amazing work that is done and yet all were of such a happy cheerful disposition.

We were treated to a display of their traditional dance and after we could talk to the children and the adults. I had the intention of sharing the TRE; somehow and in some way, this was the place to connect. I said a quick prayer. I approached one of the leaders and briefly explained what I wanted to do. He said, 'This sounds just like something we need!' He rallied nine people and we all went into a small room. In less than 40 minutes, I explained the TRE and ran through a session with them. Men and women all sat up and were truly joyful. We agreed to work together so they could start to share with their children. What followed was beyond my dreams – I had nine new recruits! We exchanged details and I left some resources. I said when back in the UK, I would teach them one way or another.

Stepping into their shoes

We then departed for the homestay. My friend and I were very lucky to be staying with Justin, who was a YODEP volunteer. I felt privileged to be able to experience the life they live. I totally wanted to be and do all that they did. No Western luxury. I embraced their sharing, helping Chikonda with the cooking and the cleaning, gaining real insight into their life. We had a long conversation in the evening. Justin said the priority for earning was food for their two children. He had started to study to become a social worker but had to stop as he could not pay the fees. Before we left, I told Justin I would pay his fees. Anything to help him step up and improve his chances for the family. Justin even taught me to make bricks! Every day when I wake up, I think of them. Beautiful people with so little, yet so much richness in their hearts.

19 months later...

On my return to the UK, I swiftly connected with those who were excited to teach. WhatsApp became the best platform. I am proud to say that I have built relationships with many in Malawi.

Chiyemkezo diligently worked with his peers and community as well as boys in the football team and in school. I sent funds for him to buy cloths for his clients as they lay on the ground. Nine months in, he coordinated the printing of T-shirts for himself and the others with me, sharing the work in Malawi. Recently, he said: *We are still doing the practice since this is the only way we can heal ourselves from the trauma that can come due to the worries of the coronavirus. I am also sharing to the others about the practice. Everyone is doing the practice at his or her home, as we observe coronavirus rules. I can never forget you, you're special to all of us in Malawi, and we are much benefiting from what you shared with us.*

YODEP

Not long after my return, I received an email from the Director of YODEP.

Dear Caroline,

We were very happy to have you at YODEP and teach some of our staff the TRE. The tool is helping the children to grow healthy and able to solve their problems as well as make good choices and decisions for their life. It is good to hear that as part of your contribution to well-being and supporting any mental health issues of our community, you are very connected to some of the small group you shared your practice with the day you came to YODEP. Thank you very much for this and on behalf of YODEP, I would like to thank you for the passion you have to serve our community.

We have children with disabilities and children infected with HIV/AIDS in our community who need a lot to be helped so that they live a happy life. The major problem is discrimination against these children, as well as their caregivers and parents. Let us stay connected and work together to help our community.

Joy Mwanda is the manager at YODEP and through him and Sarah, who was in the first group I met, they have now engaged 19 adults and between them reach out to 23 children's centres, which is incredible. One has been named TRE UK® Centre. They have taught over 4,000 children and still have a passion to share. I plan to return when I can to spend more time with them training them and to certificate those who have been sharing tirelessly with their community. Ron is going to organise things for us. The story is still being written…

Did I leave a footprint? Ania says to me often, 'Out of all us in that group, you are the only one that left something behind.' I had a vision, maybe that is why!

'I am too positive to be doubtful, too optimistic to be fearful and too determined to be defeated.'

African proverb

Caroline's Points to Ponder

1. What was the biggest challenge you ever faced?

2. Did you step up or give up?

3. Would you have climbed the mountain feeling as I did?

4. Have you left a 'footprint' or your special mark on anything? What is your legacy?

*'If we are to teach
real peace in this world,
and if we are to carry
on a real war against war,
we shall have to begin
with the children.'*

Mahatma Gandhi

Part IV - Moving Forward
Chapter Twenty
Breaking the Chains – Setting Our Children Free

I hope I have made it very clear that childhood trauma impacts on well-being in later life. I am excited because for the first time, I feel that there is hope for our children, our leaders of the future. They can learn to break the chains of holding the stress, trauma, learned behaviours and habits from their parents or guardians, and set themselves free to be who they are meant to be.

Having taught students, whether in school or at the wish of their parents, the impact is so effective. Children and teenagers have less in their Bucket, no matter what they may have experienced, than they would have 20 years later. The challenge for young people is huge, as I heard when I attended a conference on mental health and young people. When a young person has a problem, they are put in a canoe and told to keep paddling. When they fall in, they are picked up and told to keep paddling. It is not until they are virtually drowning that something finally gets done, when they are added to a waiting list to see a counsellor or therapist. However, the waiting list is so huge that often, by the time many get to their appointment they are told, 'Sorry, you are 18 now, so you have to join the adult queue!'

The power of the gatekeepers!

Seeing young people suffer is something I have come to have to accept, for if I cannot get past the gatekeepers then they have no chance. I called a Kent school having listened to the headteacher on the local radio expressing concerns about the rising anxiety of students and what little support was available for them. When I made contact to share information, why was I not surprised by the classic response, 'That sounds very interesting, I will pass it on,' and then hear no more! I know why it rarely goes anywhere – because if the one on the phone decides they do not understand, then there is an assumption no one else will, so no one and in particular, the young people in their charge, gets a chance to find out more and make a choice!

One of my biggest concerns was with University of Bristol. I was due to visit the area to teach a Workshop and was hoping to talk to the well-being officer about the Total Release Experience® with the view to talking to the students about the whole concept and impact of stress. The University of Bristol happens to have the highest student suicide rate in the country. Twice my attempts with the person in charge of Student Well-being was rejected. I would say to my team, 'What would the parents of those young people who take their own life in the future say if they were to find out that the one in charge of their child's well-being was not even willing to have a conversation? That their child was not given the chance to choose for themselves?'

There have been several more suicides since. There could have been a lot less.

So many slip through the net and go on to be very troubled adults. If only children could learn early to connect with a simple practice and engage with it as the 'thing to do' when life gets too much and build a habit. The future would look so much brighter for them and their parents or guardians.

Pete's path

Sixteen-year-old Pete found that a lot of things got to him. Exams, work, and all manner of stressful situations would make him freak out and have panic attacks, which would often stop him from sleeping, which would, in turn, make matters worse. He had tried a lot of different ways to control it but wasn't able to do so.

A family member recommended the TRE course to him.

> He shares: *I was a little unsure and a little sceptical. But I had nothing to lose and went ahead with my first session. It was a little weird to start off with but if you just go with it, it really pays off. I had positive results from week one!*

> *Having now completed the initial course, I feel totally different and I'm a lot better than I used to be with stress, anxiety and general negativity. I haven't freaked out about anything in ages. It's the best feeling in the world to be able to just get on with my life and not have to deal with all the things I've suffered with for a long, long time — especially with my GCSEs rapidly approaching and having to make choices about Sixth Form.'*

A-Level student Sally

As a 17-year-old student, Sally was dealing with the stress of work and study, which would often get the best of her and she would suffer from insomnia. Her mother had been on the TRE programme and encouraged Sally to learn herself. Without really knowing what it was, she decided that she had nothing to lose by trying it out.

> Sally shares: *I was very pleasantly surprised to notice drastic changes in my sleeping pattern shortly after beginning the sessions. I was able to sleep much more, therefore making me less tired during the day and so making me feel more energised overall.*

> *I was better able to cope with my workload and exam pressures. I know that some people may be sceptical, or may not want to try something they don't*

know, especially at my age, however I would highly recommend it because the results could truly improve your daily life as they did mine.

The prospect of a troubled future

This is the story of how 16-year-old Tony's life was turned around when he saw little prospect of that ever happening.

Tony was referred to his psychotherapist for support to manage his anxiety and other difficult feelings. He has a sister with severe mental health problems, which understandably had a significant impact on him. He had anger issues, anxiety and a general lack of motivation, that was impacting on his overall emotional well-being and his education.

Tony initially did not engage with the therapist. He was open about his ambivalence regarding counselling and needed some encouragement to trust in the therapeutic process. His goals were to feel less stressed and anxious, to sleep better and to improve motivation in support of his imminent GSCEs.

At the start of the sessions with the psychotherapist using GAD7* and PHQ-9*, Tony scored severe for depression and anxiety. He felt low and was withdrawn.

The sessions allowed him to explore his traumatic experiences, distressing thoughts and difficult feelings, and offered a space for talking and an exploration of the impact of trauma on the brain, alongside grounding strategies to help him cope. He identified feeling "numb and trapped" with an overwhelming sense of responsibility and sadness. Having attended 12 sessions and continuing to feel "stuck", Tony began to question the potential option of medication. 'What if I never feel better?' With support from his therapist, his doctor reluctantly prescribed an SSRI (antidepressant), alongside an agreed extension of therapeutic support.

Tony passed all his GCSEs and was looking forward to his new college course. However, the transition proved challenging and he continued

* *See glossary at the back for the full meaning.*

to struggle with low mood and anxiety and at times even had suicidal thoughts. He was encouraged to seek advice from his doctor and his medication was changed, alongside a safety plan and continued therapeutic support. Crucially, he attended a TRE UK® Workshop with his therapist.

Tony continued his practice at home, which he describes as 'meditation' – he notices a 'clearer' head. He is beginning to explore his creativity through drawing, and his sleep has improved. He notices that he is calmer and less irritated; his motivation at college is improving. Approaching planned discharge from the psychotherapist, he has begun to let go of his sense of responsibility for his sister and is talking positively of himself and has clear aspirations. "I couldn't see a future before and now I can."

Breakdown of assessment tool scores

	1.5.19 Start Psychotherapy	14.9.19 Review Score	27.11.19 Start of the TRE	29.1.20 8 weeks later
PHQ9	19	19	18	13
GAD7	18	18	12	6

Without the TRE session, he would have needed ongoing support in therapy which was not possible. He has now been discharged. Since learning to Release, Tony has not needed to seek advice from his GP.

There are thousands of children and teenagers across the country that are struggling with anxiety. The impact that Releasing has is swift and effective. It is a far better solution than considering the prospect of young people growing up on a diet of antidepressants. Surely our children deserve better than that? All who have influence over any child have the power to help them break the chains of their past and live an amazing life. They are our Diamonds of the future. There is nothing more heart-warming than knowing another young life has been turned around.

I have worked with children as young as five and they love to connect with the practice: unlike adults, they do not have the need to analyse or question, they just get on with it. They know it leaves them with a feel-good factor. If encouraged to do it regularly, then they will see it as the norm and integrate it into their life.

> **'We desire to bequeath two things to our children;
> the first one is roots and the other one is wings.'**
>
> *African proverb*

Caroline's Points to Ponder

1. Do you remember your own teenage worries and how you coped? Is it any different today?

2. Do you know any teenagers suffering anxiety and depression?

3. What impact do you see that having on their life?

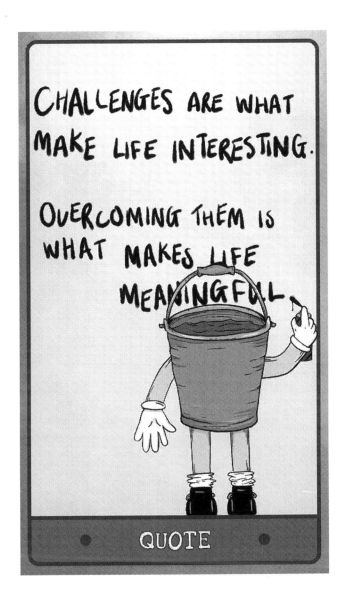

'Ignorance is always afraid of change.'

Jawaharlal Nehru
First Prime Minister of India

Chapter Twenty-One
Conclusion:
The Price of Ignorance –
Changing Mindsets –
And a Message to Leaders

In this book, I have shared a concept with you that may have gone way beyond what you thought you understood about the power of your own body, as you have discovered in all the shared stories.

Too many people lose years of their life because of ill health. Too many waste years of their life feeling angry, bitter or resentful. Too many live in isolation, too many have addictions, too many end up in prison, too many have insurmountable, physical, mental and emotional problems, and too many take their own life.

Why is this? Well I hope you are now thinking HISTORY and full BUCKETS! Time now for a new way of thinking before too many more die before their time. Before too many more children live their life carrying the scars of their childhood through to their adult life. Time now to think twice about what is really behind the reason your mother, father, brother, sister, friend or anyone else in your life behaved the way they did or still do what they do. What is behind their 'painted smile'? What happened to them which meant that they could not go on anymore?

How many more celebrities, footballers, sports personalities, politicians, business leaders and other high-profile individuals, who wear that painted smile so well, will we see suffer? How many more of them will burn out or have to leave their job because of stress and anxiety? How many more good people will take their own life? How many more unwritten and untold stories are out there of abuse, prejudice, childhood traumas, relationship issues, grief, loss, and so much more? How many more will become addicts as they try to heal themselves? They all fill their stress BUCKET as you do and like you, all have the ability to Release.

The world is changing post-COVID-19. Mindsets need to change too. We have seen during the most challenging times the world has faced in decades, that there has been an acute rise in mental health issues. NHS staff and carers, as key worker staff around the world, are experiencing stress and anxiety like never before. If we do not want to see more physical, mental and emotional ailments and illnesses, or heart attacks and strokes, if we do not want to hear about more physical attacks, murders or suicides, then mindsets **have** to change.

You have choices. You can ignore or deny the signs your body is giving you that your BUCKET is under strain, or you can make a new discovery and learn to Release. Even if you feel great now, you don't know how much better you could feel! Even if you think you have tried everything – let me tell you that you have one last thing left to try. Ironic, isn't it, that you had the answer all the time! Still not sure? Ask yourself this – 'What have I got to lose?'

Our business mentor, Sammy Blindell, told us all at a conference, 'When you know what you know, you've a DUTY to share.' Strong words, but so true. This book is about sharing what I know and I hope as a result that there will be a faster-moving ripple effect – for I fear that unless mindsets are changed, when it comes to the most precious thing we all have – our health – there are going to be some bigger problems ahead.

A Message to Leaders

'A Leader is one who knows the way,
goes the way and shows the way.'

John Maxwell
American speaker, pastor and author of
'The 21 Irrefutable Laws of Leadership'

If you are a leader, then you have such an influence on those you lead. Be they children or adults, they will look to you for support and inspiration. They look at how you behave, your language, and as an influencer on their life, they may choose you as a role model. That comes with incredible responsibility.

As I bring this book to a conclusion, I have invited leaders in their field that know the power of Releasing to share their message with you.

If just one life is saved, then this whole book will have been worth it.

To Parents

'To be in your children's memories tomorrow,
you have to be in their lives today.'

Barbara Johnson
American literary critic and translator

Hello,

My name is Daniel Wood, and with my mum Caroline, I am passionate about sharing my message to all of you parents reading this.

Over the years I have had some great insights into the amazing power of this simple, easy-to-do practice. None so great as when the penny dropped of its potential for parents as leaders.

Parenting Challenge!

Ask yourself, 'How are you leading your children in dealing with stress?' Stress or trauma is not escapable; you will have read how it negatively impacts health in many ways but is also a source of personal growth.

You have also read about all the habits that are used as a get-by strategy. So, let me ask you, 'How do you lead your children who look to you for examples to follow? Do you drink more? Eat more? Smoke more? Work or train harder? What language do you use when under stress? How do you behave? What do your children see?'

Bucking the Trend

I have three much-loved children. They have seen me embrace a great career potential and achieve success but also the consequence of failing to cope with what hit me hardest in life – divorce. They had to see me at my lowest having to deal with major financial losses and homelessness. However, they also witnessed too that despite my mistakes, I picked myself up and have kept moving forward, which I still am doing. They do not see me following the trend because I don't store my stress. The Total Release Experience®, turned my life around, for I know without it I would not be in such a great place as I am today.

I am reminded of the words of the song 'Cats in the Cradle' by Harry Chapin; perhaps you know it? The song resonated with me and I began to see it in my life: *I'm gonna be like you, Dad / You know I'm gonna be like you* And as the song ends... *He'd grown up just like me / My boy was just like me.*

I would be very happy now for my boy (and girls) to grow up just like me!

Parenting Opportunity!

I recognised that teaching my children what I know was one of the best gifts I could ever give them. I cannot protect them from what life will throw at them, for like all of us, it is their individual journey. What I can give them though is a life tool, so that unlike me and all of you, they will not carry their stress and traumatic experiences into their adult life. They have a choice to use this life tool and I know they do. As they Release, I know the chains will be broken and they will shine through to be the special Diamonds they are, not just to me, but the world in which they live.

Do you remember reading Darren's story? He was the client who took off with his family in their camper van to have an adventure. He has something else to share:

> *I fully agree with Daniel with regards to reaching an understanding about the power of releasing with your children. Releasing is such a valuable tool for children – I can only imagine how useful it will be when life throws challenges at them in years to come; when they take their first exams, driving tests, have important relationships and so on.*

> *At times in the past, I have felt pressure to encourage my children to Release on a regular basis, which seems ironic, but together, my wife and I realised that we simply needed to model the behaviour we wanted them to see, much in the same way we do in other areas of our parenting. In order for it to be fully embedded into our family routine, we must take a more holistic approach. We dropped the idea that we always needed to escape into a quiet room to do our Releasing, and now we just embrace it, making it more accessible for everyone. There are days now too that my seven-year-old will say, 'Dad, I think you need to empty your Bucket!'*

Unless you are prepared to lead the way for your children – who else is going to? I invite you to join the growing number of parents leading their children and to start leading yours with much more than learning to cope. To follow your lead and together 'shake it off', so they can thrive and shine in a challenging and changing world.

Daniel

**'The sign of great parenting is not the child's behaviour.
The sign of truly great parenting is the parent's behaviour.'**

Andy Smithson
American psychotherapist, social worker, author,
speaker and father

To Boarding School Staff

'Teachers affect eternity;
no one can ever tell where their influence stops.'

Henry Brook Adams
American historian, journalist and political writer.

Hello,

My name is Jennifer Norman. As an experienced and passionate housemistress at a boarding school, I have supported both boys and girls with many mental health problems ranging from eating disorders, self-harm, depression, anxiety, anger outbursts and psychosis. These young people experience a vast number of challenges each and every day. They are away from their family for long periods of time, some may have gone through the separation or divorce of their parents, bereavement of a loved one or pet, identity confusions, academic pressures, friendship troubles, bullying... the list continues. It is daunting being a teenager.

My priority has been to offer a range of interventions to help support students at these challenging times. Whilst I was reflecting on the range of interventions on offer, I began to ponder the thought that I needed to support both myself and my staff, as well as the students, by becoming more attuned to our own emotional well-being. My key starting point was not the students but my staff; if we were more aware of our own stressors or even better at managing them, we could better support and model positive behaviours in this area.

The key is to get everyone to talk more openly about their ups and downs; stress is normal and difficult to avoid in modern society: if we can't support ourselves, how can we be offering the best care to our students? This got me thinking.

It was time to step outside the comfort zone, while thinking outside the box, and take a risk to widen the intervention offering. The TRE was offered to our staff and students. It was good for staff to empty their Stress Bucket to help with the work life balance, but most of all, they could reassure students that this was an important life tool that would be vital as they went through life. It would help them at challenging times in their lives beyond their time in school, such as exams, driving test, new jobs, meeting new people, and so on. After the TRE course, our students notably improved grades and were happier in themselves as their anxiety lifted.

For me, this is an excellent programme that I offer my students. Not all of them want to talk, but they do want to offload the pressures – Release from the TRE allows this. The prospect of all schools supporting the physical, mental and emotional health of staff and pupils, would be such a positive step to massively reduce the growing problem of anxiety in young people. I would recommend to all headteachers and well-being managers in all schools (not just boarding schools) to consider the benefits of offering something so simple, powerful, cost-effective and practical for all in your care.

Jennifer
Housemistress and teacher

'We educators stand at a special point in time.'

Robert J. Marzano
American author and educational specialist

To Educational Leaders

'If you are a leader, do everything you can to grow yourself and create the right environment for others to grow.'
Law 6: Law of Environment

John C. Maxwell
Author of 'The 15 Invaluable Laws of Growth'

Hello

My name is Lelia Berkeley, and I have been in primary education for over 30 years, with 22 years as a headteacher in three different schools. I am also a Special Needs Coordinator and an Attachment Lead, having been trained by Louise Bomber. My passion has always been for child-centred education, firmly rooted in child psychology and developmental theory. I have been acutely aware throughout my career of how important educators are in supporting children and families who have experienced trauma of one form or another. I have worked with psychologists, doctors, therapists and social workers to coordinate much needed social and mental health support and I have learnt so much from them.

At this current time leading a school through the COVID-19 pandemic, this aspect of our work in schools has quite rightly taken priority. Well-being for staff and pupils has never been higher on the educational agenda. As an Attachment Lead, I am aware of how important relationships are in supporting recovery and of the links between mind and body and how we store trauma within us. The influences of neuroscience in shaping our understanding of trauma is widely acknowledged and this message is slowly finding its way into schools. However, we remain 'time poor' in introducing new approaches into school and embedding cultural change. We often rely on key people leading on new initiatives and roll-outs and there remains much inequality in what children receive in relation to supportive strategies in schools. We are very much in need of a more universal approach where staff can be trained easily and can experience change for themselves. From this informed and knowledgeable position, they can then cascade training to a class of children. They will provide children with a tool for well-being.

This tool will be powerful in that it will be for life. It will be easily accessible, and the children can choose to use it to help them feel better and deal with stress. This does not mean that children cannot benefit from other means of support in schools, it just means that there is a universal offer for all. Some children will require 'top-ups' from other modalities as part of a personalised well-being programme and will be better placed to access this support with a calmer sensory system. It would be great if we could encourage parents to learn too. Parents are in a strong position to be fully involved at this time due to their valuable contribution in supporting home-learning programmes during the pandemic.

As the headteacher of a school that promotes a bespoke and holistic approach to supporting vulnerable children, I think it is great that there is the Total Release Experience® option to build resilience for all. I also cannot stress enough how important it is that we prioritise the well-being of school staff at this time. TRE UK® does, I believe, offer a timely solution for current times. I am excited to be part of a pilot project bringing the TRE to my school. I see this approach as addressing the missing piece of the jigsaw in supporting pupil well-being in schools. We now have an approach that addresses the physiological dimension of trauma which is often talked about, but without the practical solution.

Lelia
St Andrew's Primary School
Marks Tey, Essex

'What you want to do is get people from having a fear of change to a fear of what will happen if we don't change.'

Bryan Goodwin
President and CEO of McREL International,
non-profit education research and development organization,
author, former teacher and journalist.

To the Service Sector

'Courage is not the absence of fear,
but rather the judgement that something else
is more important than fear.'

Ambrose Redmoon
American author and band manager

Hello,

My name is Paul Harris. I have been a serving police officer in various forces throughout the UK. In my twenty years of service, to date I have been exposed to trauma and stress of varying degrees. As a young 22-year-old officer I can still recall to this day the first time I saw someone die because they had been stabbed, and the impact it had on me and my family. Back then, the well-being of an officer was not really a headline consideration. It may well have been an afterthought, a tick box exercise, but generally the consensus was that we are 'duty-bound' to understand why someone has died and what can we do about it to bring about justice, support to bereaved families and reduce impact on communities.

For many years as an officer, I myself am confident to say within a work setting, 'That incident was very tough for me'. As with many people, I felt that as a front line service, it was part of my duty and my pride to say, 'I'm OK,' even when I was not. But like most people in my position, you find ways to cope, be it reading, fitness or walking a dog: there is some method to release that stress, or empty that bucket… For me it was running and fitness, and this was a big baseline release that had to be part of my everyday living. If the running stopped, the stress built up, and the issues became evident to all that were close to me.

In 2017 serious stress factors both at work and at home overtook me physically and mentally to the point that a one-mile run felt like I was dragging a tank behind me. The harder I pushed, the worse I ran; the stress grew more and the burden of failure mentally and physically hit me. What was once a release through running, became a prison of torture and pain. On reflection now, the cycle of doom was all-consuming, and if I hadn't found something, I am unsure what the outcome would have been for me. In 2019, still not coping, I was diagnosed with inflammatory bowel disease and through the luck of the gods I found a GP that seemed to understand my level and that I needed another option.

At that time, I was not a person who wanted to talk to people about my problems; I wanted a solution that I could take responsibility for, and that's when the Total Release Experience® was introduced in my life. That day changed my perspective on many things and the TRE was the additional outlet that gave me time to change my mindset to have strength to be able to say, 'It's OK not to be OK!'

I cannot advocate enough the effects that 'shaking it out' can have on an individual. I practice twice a week in the comfort of my own home, and it's a massive benefit to me.

My vision and plan are to see the TRE embedded in front line services, as 20 years ago, at that first murder, it would have been a welcome tool in my box to help me cope. Luckily now, in 2020, front line services are becoming more open to alternative methods of stress release. As a leader, if you are reading this and see any hint of self-reflection in what I have written, you owe it to yourself and others to try this…

Paul

'A noble leader answers not to the trumpet calls of self-promotion, but to the hushed whispers of necessity.'

Mollie Marti
American psychologist, lawyer, researcher, humanitarian and author of 'Walking with Justice'

To Business Leaders

'Leadership is not a matter of authority;
it is a matter of influence.
A true leader teaches others to understand more,
motivates them to be more and
inspires them to become more.'

Michael Josephson
Former law professor and attorney

Hello,

My name is Sammy Blindell and I am an Entrepreneurial Global Brand Builder and Business Leader. There has never been a more critical time in history for you to step up than now. The world needs a trusted, credible leader like you to take the lead and shine like the true lighthouse you are, beaming with all the integrity and credibility that you have worked so hard to build throughout your entire career. But as Caroline has mentioned several times throughout this book, with leadership comes great responsibility and that responsibility must be to ourselves before anyone else.

'But I don't have time to put myself first,' I hear you say.

Yes, I said that too, until I worked so hard that I burned out, became seriously ill through stress, and ended up in hospital four times in just over three months with suspected heart attacks. I eventually walked away from my £7.8 million business – leaving behind everything and everyone I knew so I could get my health back. Only after many months of recuperation did I truly understand that I should have put my 'self' and my health before anything else, because without it I lost everything anyway.

The Dalai Lama, when asked what surprised him most about humanity, said:

> *Man. Because he sacrifices his health in order to make money. Then he sacrifices money to recuperate his health. And then he is so anxious about the future that he does not enjoy the present; the result being that he does not live in the present or the future; he lives as if he is never going to die, and then dies having never really lived.*

This quote spoke directly to me and maybe it speaks to you too. I never want you to tread the unnecessary path that I took before I burned out.

I spent 13 years in branding and marketing before launching my first business in 2002. I went on to build six more companies in the business growth sector and after 12 years of relentless drive to make millions of pounds, dollars and euros for my clients, I badly burned out and walked away with nothing. Please don't let this be you.

As a successful serial entrepreneur, I didn't want to leave the world of business behind. However, I knew that if I was going to stay in the world of Brand Leadership, I had to start looking after myself.

Putting myself first used to be an alien concept to me and I still have moments when I have to remind myself about it! But I have never been happier, more productive, more energized, more connected, more focused and more free than I am now. My wish for you is to take action on the incredible advice you are getting in Caroline's book so that you too can be free to be an inspirational, influential leader by being the best you can be. This can only happen when you let go of the negative aspects of stress.

With love and blessings,
Sammy xx

'The future depends on what we do in the present.'
Mahatma Gandhi

I am so grateful for those who are supporting our mission, leading the way and sharing for the benefit of others.

Together, we can make a difference!

'Growth is never by mere chance;
it is the result of forces working together.'
James Cash Penney
American businessman and entrepreneur

Caroline's Points to Ponder

1. Whom do you lead?

2. Are you inspired to lead others towards a brighter, healthier future?

3. Will you take any action now?

*'The natural healing force
within each of us is
the greatest force in getting well.'*

*Hippocrates
Greek physician*

Chapter Twenty-Two
The Last Word –
A Doctor's Perspective and
Her Message to Leaders

I had a phone call one day and was quite excited once the call was over. I said to Daniel, 'That was Dr Alison Graham from Yaxley, looking to find out more about our work. I said we would be delighted to arrange a Workshop for her and a few others as she was keen to experience the practice.' I will let Alison take up the story and deliver her message.

Hello,

My name is Alison Graham and I am a GP partner with over 30 years of post-graduate clinical experience. I have always found the mind-body connection fascinating and in Primary Care there is abundant opportunity to see that powerful dynamic in action. We see a huge amount of ill-health due to issues that begin with the brain, resulting in an overflow of toxic feelings, but end up causing physical symptoms. Early in my career it was frustrating that even though I was becoming skilled at identifying what was wrong, it also became clear that the tool kit I had at my disposal to treat these patients was completely inadequate. Drugs or a long wait for 'talking therapy' was about it for treatment and for prevention? Even less.

I have spent decades looking for the answer to prevent and treat my own stress and that of my patients. I explored hypnosis with Paul McKenna, NLP (Neuro-Linguistic Programming) with founder Richard Bandler, and looked at techniques both inside and outside the medical arena such as

TFT Tapping*, Havening* and EMDR. All were fascinating, helped me and quite a few patients along the way, but all required a lot of trained clinical input. I searched for techniques that were accessible as soon as the need arose, inexpensive and most importantly, empowered the patient to be the master of their health. This autonomy, I believe, is essential.

I read many books about how trauma affects people. Two that resonated the most with me were *Trauma: From Lockerbie to 7/7* by Professor Gordon Turnbull and the classic *The Body Keeps the Score* by one of the world's leading authorities on the subject, Bessel van der Kolk. Both spoke of how trauma is trapped like a neurological scar in the body, a connection to the past and that pathology and disease are caused by that scar echoing over and over. Gordon sums trauma up in a nutshell: *it is not possible to talk it out of the body*. Had van der Kolk's book been written today, I wonder if his final chapter would talk about TRE as he gets so close to it!

I stumbled across Caroline and TRE UK® quite by accident. I am Chair of a charity called Young People's Counselling Service (YPCS) which provides high-quality counselling to fill the huge gap in NHS services. A friend of an ex-trustee heard of the technique and thought that we might be interested. It sounded too good to be true. It was surely impossible that the answer could be so simple. I went to the Workshop with a colleague who is a psychologist. Both of us went with an open mind but also a healthy dose of scepticism and not at all expecting to get the results that we did.

Do I know how it works? Not really. I always quip that there is much in medicine we use routinely that remains a mystery and that we use our smart phones happily unaware of how they operate! *Does it help everything in everybody all the time?* No but what does? It certainly has a greater success rate than most drugs I prescribe. *Is it safe?* Caroline has over eight years of experience and no adverse effects have been noted, although the emotional Release can be powerful and occasionally temporarily overwhelming. It is important therefore that people are taught properly how to do this and how to manage the Release afterwards.

* *See glossary at the back for the full meaning.*

There seems to be noticeable effects during and immediately after a Release. I cried the first time – no idea why – and felt so relaxed I could have fallen asleep. The relaxation was very deep. There are also things that happen between sessions which is why regular practice is best. It is spring cleaning for the brain, removing old clutter and ensuring that new stresses don't take hold. Chronic stress is the cause of the majority of illness that I see on a daily basis and there is mounting evidence to show that it causes measurable inflammation in the body. This in turn results not only in symptoms but recognisable diseases such as colitis, rheumatoid arthritis and some cancers. Conditions characterised by central pain sensitivity problems, such as fibromyalgia, simply didn't seem to exist when I started in Primary Care, yet we now have increasing numbers. Many sufferers are now on addictive opiates, sleeping tablets and other drugs that work on the nervous system like Pregabalin.

Are they better on this toxic and expensive poly-pharmacy? I would argue not really. By focusing on prescribing only for the crippling pain they feel and not looking for the root causes, I think we are doing them a great injustice. *Would the TRE help them?* There is lots of inspiring anecdotal evidence, but clinical trials are always needed if we expect the NHS to spare some resources. The TRE is, however, supported by a local pain consultant which gives me hope that wider acceptance will come in time as it did for EMDR. They recommended it saying that 'it fits with the bio-psychological model of pain'. However, as Gordon Turnbull says in his book, when trying out EMDR at a time when it was still considered to be akin to witchcraft (it is now offered by the NHS, by the way!), people suffer and die whilst trials are considered, run and evaluated. There has to be a balance.

In a few months, COVID-19 has swept across the world and changed the way we live for ever. Aside from pulverising economies, devastating communities, and stressing health services, it is now emerging that the long-term physical and psychological effects are only just beginning to show. **#LongCovidSOS** is a group trying to raise awareness and lobby for rehabilitation and support. Survivors in their thousands are suffering and we don't know yet the best way to help them. Those on the front line caring for patients in such huge numbers are also suffering the psychological effects of the pandemic. Months of treating this deadly virus that ravages the body in catastrophic new ways, caring for people dying apart from their families, and looking after colleagues who were critically ill, has ripped through our front line workers' emotional reserves.

Many of them are now suffering from stress, anxiety, depression, PTSD and the lesser known condition of *'moral injury'*. Moral injury most often occurs when a person commits, fails to prevent, or witnesses an act that is anathema to their moral beliefs. Who could have guessed that even the widely adopted lifesaving technique of ventilating patients on their stomachs would be so emotionally hard. I heard a clinician say that she had nightmares of bodies with no faces.

Our beleaguered mental health services chronically starved of investment simply will not cope with the numbers that will need support to recover. We owe these people more than that. Perhaps the TRE taught online might provide part of the solution. It can be deployed to the masses quickly and cheaply and once learnt, does not need expensive clinicians to maintain. How therefore can it be ignored? I ask those able to make these decisions, what is stopping you from taking a look? Perhaps run some pilot studies? Why not give it a try? These carers cannot wait years for mountains of trial data and if there is one thing that the pandemic taught many sectors, including health, it is that we can make successful, quick, positive, pragmatic and highly impactful decisions when we have to.

So, what clinical outcomes from the TRE do I see? I have seen it improve back pain after many surgeries and reduce a patient's Tramadol dose by 70%. I have seen it allow someone stuck in an aberrant grief reaction move on after 20 years where all traditional therapy had failed her. I have seen it allow a young person stuck in a dysfunctional home environment be discharged from counselling, manage his own feelings and succeed at school.

Once learnt, the TRE is self-administered, requires no clinical input and can be used in large groups. It requires no special equipment and transcends language barriers. It is available online now for a small fee. However, it should be available 'on prescription', taught at school and available free for all our COVID-19 traumatised health and social care workers. There is no need for a 'tsunami of PTSD', as the Royal College of Psychiatrists is predicting. There is simply not enough skilled resource available even if the mental health budget was doubled. We need to look at more innovative options.

I encourage every leader (whomever you lead) to have a look, try it for yourself and take a tiny chance. Then you will see what all the fuss is about. This technique is a game-changer.

Dr Alison Graham

'The greatest medicine of all is teaching people how not to need it.'

Hippocrates
Greek physician

Connecting with Alison was one of those meant-to-be moments. She is rare amongst doctors, with her open mind, her support for our work, but more importantly, for leading by her own example, supporting her patients, knowing they too can heal themselves.

Caroline's Points to Ponder

1. Would your doctor be open to Alison's advice?

2. If your doctor offered you either a prescription for anxiety or suggested you learned to Release, which would you take?

'Faith is moving forward even when things don't make sense, trusting that in hindsight... everything will become clear.'

Mandy Hale
New York Times best-selling author of 'The Single Woman'

Afterword

Thank you for reading this book. It was a challenge selecting the stories; I have so many. I hope you feel awakened to the idea that you have something more to discover about yourself and your ability to Release.

Can you imagine a world of Buckets, transformed to Diamonds? What a happy, peaceful, grounded, and more productive world it would be!

Daniel and I have total faith in the power of the human body to heal.

It is a practice for all the reasons you have read about, including those of you who are also:

- Curious
- Wanting to come off medication
- Looking to get off their addictions
- About to give up on ever getting better
- Prepared to take back control and responsibility

Of course, it is not a panacea for all ills, especially if dis-ease has gone too far, but even then peace can be found. I hope this book has sparked some curiosity and excitement in you such that when you think you have tried everything, you now know that there is one more thing to try!

Whether you are intrigued, think it is a load of nonsense or perhaps even 'snake oil', you are entitled to your opinion. All I ask is that you make your judgement based on experience. I know if I had walked away from my first clients and not discovered from my own experience and self-practice, if I had judged it before engaging with it, there would be less Diamonds in the world than are out there shining now in a way they never thought possible.

For everyone who has healed from their past, for those now standing up for themselves and speaking out, for those who got to the brink and managed to step back, and for those leading the way with their example and inspiring others with their story – to coin Tom's phrase, as 'Sergeant Major' Purvey, I salute you all!

P.S.

- Marcus has been in touch and he has stayed out of prison longer than he ever has done. He took himself to rehab to be totally clean. When his employer learned he was an ex-offender, he was dismissed. But don't you and I know something about him now that they don't?!

- Darren and his family have set off again to pick up where they left off, to live more of the dream.

- Mary is still discovering more and loving the journey.

As for TRE UK® …

My journey is far from over as we continue to grow, for there is still much to do. At the close of one of my first Workshops in Brighton, a lady suggested, 'You need special people to do this with you.' That has resonated with me ever since. Back in 2012, I wrote my own training programme and was proud that it was Accredited by the Federation of Holistic Therapists. It is, and remains to be, the only externally accredited course of its kind, both nationally and internationally.

Jayne, Carly and Sally continue to be patient and supportive practitioners, as Daniel and I in the light of COVID-19 have yet again been developing and creating on all levels so we can now reach out globally. They are special ladies, who are as excited as we are about the way forward. We shall be looking for more 'special people' before too long. Just as the world changes, so do we and that is exciting!

*'A year from now
you will wish you had
started today.'*
Karen Lamb
Author of Thea Astley: Inventing Her Own Weather

Glossary

ACEs	Adverse Childhood Experiences
Bucket	Reference to 'Stress Bucket' which we all have.
CBT	Cognitive Behaviour Therapy
CPTSD	Complex Post-Traumatic Stress Disorder
Diamond	References the Diamond that starts to shine from within when a baby is born into the world.
EMDR	Eye Movement Desensitization and Reprocessing
GAD7	Anxiety Test Questionnaire
Havening	The simple technique known as Havening, can help reduce anxiety and depression by altering the way memories are stored or recalled.
OCD	Obsessive-Compulsive Disorder
PD	Personality Disorder
PHQ-9	Depression Test Questionnaire

Psoas Muscle	The psoas muscle is located in the lower lumbar region of the spine and extends through the pelvis to the femur.
Release(ing)	Step 3 of the 5-Step Programme
Roller Coaster	Reference to the healing journey that can be challenging.
Somatisation	Is characterised by an extreme focus on physical symptoms — such as pain or fatigue.
TAP	**T**houghtfully **A**ctivate your **P**soas. The **TAP** on your Bucket.
TFT Tapping	Thought Field Therapy - utilises the meridian points and bilateral stimulation with a gentle tapping procedure.
Total Release Experience®	The 5 Step programme taught by TRE UK®
The TRE	The Total Release Experience® 5-Step Programme
TRE UK®	The Organisation
Tremoring Response	The body is encouraged to return back to a state of balance. It helps the body release deep muscular patterns of stress, tension, and trauma.

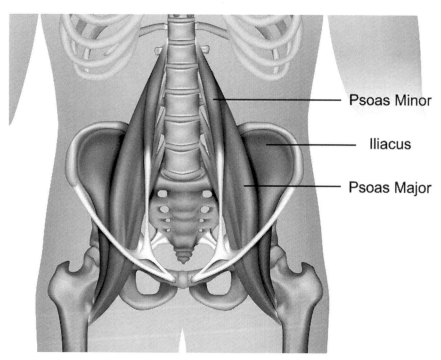

Psoas Minor

Iliacus

Psoas Major

The Psoas Muscle - The Best Kept Secret

Inspired Reading

This book was never intended to be an academic read. I therefore share the books that inspire me and influence my thinking even if not directly referenced in this book.

Books

Bourke, Joanna, *The Story of Pain: From Prayer to Painkillers*, Oxford University Press, 2014

Ellerby, Jonathan H, *Inspiration Deficit Disorder: The No-Pill Prescription To End High Stress, Low Energy, And Bad Habits*, Hay House, 2010

Gerhardt, Sue, *The Selfish Society: How We All Forgot to Love One Another and Made Money Instead*, Simon & Schuster, 2011

Levine, Peter., *Waking the Tiger: Healing Trauma*, North Atlantic Books, 1997

Maté, Dr Gabor, *When the Body Says No: The Cost of Hidden Stress*, Vermilion, 2019

Turnbull, Professor Gordon, *Trauma: From Lockerbie to 7/7*, Transworld Publishers, 2011

Sapolsky Robert M., *Why Zebras Don't Get Ulcers*, St. Martin's Press, 2004

Van der Kolk, Bessel, *The Body Keeps the Score*, Penguin, 2015

Music

Chapin, Harry, *Cats in The Cradle*, WC Music Corp., 1974

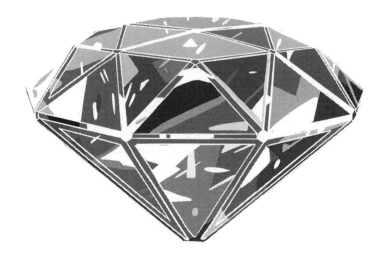

'You can't go back and change the beginning, but you can start where you are and change the ending'

C.S. Lewis
Author

About the Author

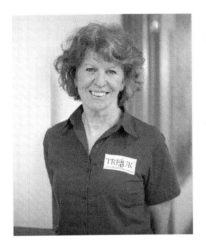

Caroline Purvey MA (Ed) is an inspirational, transformational leader and co-author of No 1 international best-selling books *Notes to My Younger Self* and *The Law of Brand Attraction*. Her life journey has led her to embark on a mission and share her passion. Leading those suffering physically, mentally and emotionally to find a new freedom from the pain of their past, Caroline's work evolved through experience and she is now the expert in her particular field, combining her unique skills and experiences from business, teaching and therapy. She also has over 25 years of yoga teaching experience with a key interest in anatomy. She is motivational, compassionate, and spiritual, and in 2019 was voted one of the Top Ten women to watch in well-being in *About Time* magazine. She is driven to reach out globally with her message, that the answer to real inner peace and freedom from pain is inside us all.

www.treuk.com
caroline@treuk.com

I hope you have enjoyed reading this book.
If you would like to leave a review on Amazon or Goodreads
and want to learn the Total Release Experience® programme,
please send a link to your review to caroline@treuk.com
and claim your discount voucher.

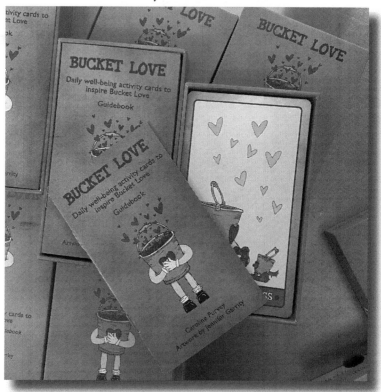

BUCKET LOVE Cards
If you liked the images found in this book,
they are taken from our inspirational pack of
31 Daily Activity Cards for well-being.
Available from www.treuk.com

You can also book our Total Release Experience® programme
by visiting our website: